Knee Stabilization

Erin Hughes, MSPT, C-PT

DSWFitness   Tucson, Arizona

A special thanks to our course reviewers.

Lenela Glass-Godwin, MS
Aqua Instructor
Tallassee Rehab
Tallassee, AL

Christy Rusdal, MS
Physical Therapist
St. Peter's Hospital
Helena, MT

Sandra Hilton, PT, CMT
Physical Therapist/Owner
Healing in Motion
Ann Arbor, MI

Cheri Tatem
Exercise Rehab Therapist
Strength Insight/Body Wisdom for Women
Boulder, CO

Managing Editor and Text Designer: Karen Thomas
Copyeditor: Monica Markley
Cover Designer: Rae Anik

ISBN-13: 978-0-9800062-3-0
ISBN-10: 0-9800062-3-6

Unconditional Guarantee
If you are not completely satisfied with the DSWFitness correspondence course *Knee Stabilization,* you may exchange your course or receive a full refund, less shipping and handling charges. Materials must be returned unmarked and intact to our office within 30 days of receiving them. All refunds will be made in the same payment method as received.

Disclaimer
DSWFitness educational products are informational only. The data and information contained in DSWFitness educational products are based upon information from various published as well as unpublished sources and merely represent general training, exercise, and health literature and practices as summarized by the authors and editors. Care has been taken to confirm the accuracy of the information presented and to describe generally accepted practice. However, the author and publisher are not responsible for errors or omissions or for any consequences from application of the information in the educational products. As publisher and distributor of educational products DSWFitness makes no guarantees or warranties, express or implied, regarding the currentness, completeness, or scientific accuracy of this information, nor does the publisher/ distributor guarantee or warrant the fitness, marketability, efficacy, or accuracy of this information for any particular purpose. Information from unpublished sources, books, research journals, and articles is not intended to replace the advice or attention of medical or healthcare professionals. This summary is also not intended to direct anyone's behavior or replace anyone's independent professional judgment. If you have a problem with your health, before you embark on any health, fitness, or sports training program, including the programs herein, please seek advice and clearance from a qualified medical or healthcare professional. The publishers have made every effort to trace the copyright holders for borrowed material. If they have inadvertently overlooked any, they will be pleased to make necessary arrangements at the first opportunity.

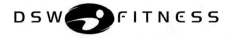

CENTER FOR CONTINUING EDUCATION

602 E. ROGER RD • TUCSON, AZ 85705 • 520.292.0011 • FAX 520.292.0066 • EXAMS@DSWFITNESS.COM • WWW.DSWFITNESS.COM

Contents

History of ACL Reconstruction Surgery 85
Previous Knee Injury 87

Appendix: PEP Program 91

About the Author 115

Knee Anatomy and Biomechanics

The knee joint is the largest joint in the body. It is a complex joint that relies on a number of muscles and supporting structures for stability. Proper function and stability of the knee joint is essential for weight bearing and the ability to ambulate. Understanding the anatomy and biomechanics of the knee joint facilitates the development of a safe and efficient exercise program for clients to improve the strength and stability of the knee. This chapter outlines the anatomy of the knee and describes the movements and mechanics specific to this joint.

Knee Joint

The knee joint is also referred to as the *tibiofemoral joint* because it is formed by the distal end of the femur and the proximal end of the tibia. The convex, or rounded, condyles of the femur sit in the concavity of the tibial plateau. The knee joint is classified as a hinge joint, which allows motion in primarily one plane. Although the two greatest movements of the knee are flexion and extension, the joint also allows for some slight rotation. Other examples of hinge joints are the elbow and the ankle.

A strong membranous capsule surrounds the joint and keeps it bathed in nourishing and protective synovial fluid. This capsule is very extensive, making the knee's synovial cavity the largest joint space in the body. On either end of the femur and the tibia is a layer of cartilage that serves as cushioning for the joint and allows for shock absorption between the bones.

The other important articulation of the knee is the patellofemoral joint. This joint is formed by the patella, or kneecap, and the femur. The function of the patellofemoral joint is to increase the mechanical advantage of the quadriceps muscles and allow greater force generation across the knee. When the knee is flexed and extended, the patella moves within the patellofemoral groove of the femur. The patella can also rotate and tilt, depending on the pull of the muscles and tendons surrounding the joint. The underside of the patella is covered with some of the thickest cartilage in the human body. This cartilage minimizes friction and helps the patella glide smoothly along the femur.

Although the fibula is not considered to be part of the knee joint itself, there are muscles and ligaments that insert on this bone that help to produce movement at the knee.

Knee Kinematics

Kinematics is the study of motion in the body. The main motions occurring at the knee joint are flexion and extension. Flexion and extension are two terms used to describe anatomic movement of the body. Flexion is defined as bending, or decreasing, the angle between two bony segments, while extension is the straightening, or increasing, the angle between the body parts. In regards to rotation, medial rotation occurs when the lower leg or tibia turns inward. Lateral rotation is described as the tibia turning outward on the femur.

Varus and valgus are two additional terms that are similar to abduction and adduction at the joint. They are not normal physiologic movements at the knee joint but are important to discuss because they describe deformities of the knee and the direction of motion that may cause injury. Varus occurs when the distal segment (the tibia) is deviated medially with respect to the proximal segment (the femur). On the other hand, valgus alignment occurs when the distal segment (the tibia) is deviated laterally with respect to the proximal segment (the femur). Clients with excessive valgus of their knees are also described as having "knock knees," while those with varus deformities are considered to be bowlegged. One other type of knee deformity occurs when one or both of the knees are in hyperextension. This is also referred to as genu recurvatum.

Knee Biomechanics

As the knee moves into full extension in a standing position, a rotational movement occurs in which the femur rotates medially in relation to the tibia. This motion is involuntary and is due to the size differences in the femoral condyles. The medial condyle is larger and continues to roll into extension even after the lateral condyle has stopped and becomes the pivot for the rotation. Increasing tension in the ligaments may also contribute to this rotational movement. Some texts refer to this physiological motion as the "screw-home mechanism," or "locking mechanism," because the knee is considered to be locked into full extension at this moment.

To "unlock" the joint and flex the knee, the reverse motion must occur. When standing, the femur must laterally rotate on the tibia before the knee can be fully flexed. The popliteus muscle plays a role in initiating this movement. Damage to the joint can occur if the unlocking motion does not occur prior to flexing the knee.

Knee Muscles

The muscles surrounding the knee are some of the strongest and longest muscles in the body. They are very important for producing flexion and extension movement at the knee but are also essential for maintaining the stability of the joint.

Anterior Knee Muscles

The quadriceps are the largest group of muscles around the knee and function primarily to extend the joint. These muscles also act to slow knee flexion motion. For example, the quadriceps are active not only during activities such as climbing stairs but also work to control your descent when walking down a steep hill.

The quadriceps are divided into four separate muscles. Each of the muscles insert on the proximal aspect of the patella and to the tibial tuberosity through the patellar ligament.

Rectus femoris   Originates on the anterior aspect of the ilium on the hip and inserts on the patella and tibia. *Action on the knee:* Extends the knee.

Vastus medialis   Originates on the proximal femur and inserts on the patella and tibia. *Action on the knee:* Extends the knee.

Vastus lateralis   Originates on the proximal femur and inserts on the patella and tibia. *Action on the knee:* Extends the knee.

Vastus intermedius   Originates on the anterior femur and inserts on the patella and tibia. *Action on the knee:* Extends the knee.

Posterior Knee Muscles

The hamstring muscles are located on the posterior aspect of the knee and act to bend or move the knee into flexion. The hamstrings are divided into three separate muscles.

Biceps femoris   Originates on the ischium of the hip and the proximal aspect of the femur and inserts on the head of the fibula and lateral tibia. *Action on the knee:* Flexes and laterally rotates the knee.

Semitendinosus   Originates on the ischium of the hip and inserts on the medial tibia. *Action on the knee:* Flexes and medially rotates the knee.

Semimembranosus   Originates on the ischium of the hip and inserts on the medial tibia. *Action on the knee:* Flexes and medially rotates the knee.

Additional Knee Muscles

The remaining muscles all act to flex the knee joint but insert on different aspects of the tibia. The pes anserinus (meaning *goose's foot*) is a group of muscle tendons that insert on the proximal medial tibia. From anterior to posterior, these three muscles are the sartorius, gracilis, and the semitendinosus. The pes anserinus, along with the tendon of the semimembranosus, help prevent abnormal valgus and excess lateral rotation of the joint.

Sartorius   Originates on the anterior aspect of the ilium and inserts on the medial tibia. *Action on the knee:* Flexes and medially rotates the knee. The sartorius is the longest muscle in the human body.

Gracilis   Originates on the pubic bone and inserts on the medial tibia. *Action on the knee:* Flexes and medially rotates the knee.

Popliteus   Originates on the lateral femur and inserts on the proximal posterior aspect of the tibia. *Action on the knee:* Flexes and rotates the knee.

Gastrocnemius   Originates on the posterior aspect of the medial and lateral femur and inserts into the posterior calcaneus via the Achilles tendon. *Action on the knee:* Flexes the knee.

Knee Supporting Structures

The other supporting structures of the knee consist of the ligaments, menisci, and bursae. Along with increasing the joint's stability, these structures assist in shock absorption and reducing friction.

Ligaments

There are four main ligaments in the knee that are essential in providing multidirectional stability to the joint. The cruciate ligaments control the back-and-forth motion of the knee while the collateral ligaments limit the sideways movement. The anterior cruciate and posterior cruciate ligaments are located within the joint capsule and prevent excess

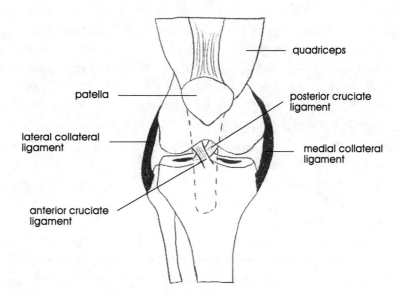

quadriceps

patella

posterior cruciate
ligament

lateral collateral
ligament

medial collateral
ligament

anterior cruciate
ligament

Figure 1.1. Knee joint

rotation and translation of the bones. They are named the cruciate ligaments because they cross on the inside of the joint, resembling the letter *x*. The term *cruciate* comes from the Latin word *crux,* which means *cross.*

The collateral ligaments are another set of ligaments that are important for the stability of the knee. The medial collateral and lateral collateral ligaments are located on either side of the knee joint and prevent excess sidebending, or varus and valgus, stress on the knee. Figure 1.1 illustrates the knee joint and the four main ligaments.

Anterior cruciate ligament (ACL)   Runs upward and laterally from the anterior tibia to the lateral femoral condyle. The ligament becomes tight when the knee is extended and slack when the knee is flexed. *Action:* Prevents excessive forward movement of the tibia on the femur (tibial translation), limits rotation, and prevents hyperextension of the knee. Without the ACL, the knee becomes susceptible to degeneration. Injury to this ligament is quite common, especially in sports that require quick stopping, turning, or contact with other players.

Posterior cruciate ligament (PCL)   Runs upward and medially from the posterior tibia to the medial femoral condyle. The ligament becomes tight when the knee is flexed. *Action:* Prevents excessive backward movement of the tibia on the femur and hyperflexion of the knee. The posterior cruciate ligament is stronger than the anterior cruciate ligament and is injured less often.

Medial collateral ligament (MCL)   Runs from the medial condyle of the femur to the tibia. A deeper portion of the ligament also attaches to the medial meniscus. *Action:* Prevents excessive valgus from widening the medial aspect of the joint. Also helps restrain lateral rotation of the tibia. This ligament becomes tight when the knee is extended and slack when the knee is flexed. Injuries to the MCL often result in simultaneous damage to the medial meniscus due to their attachment to one another.

Lateral collateral ligament (LCL)   Runs beneath the tendon of the biceps femoris muscle from the lateral condyle of the femur to the head of the fibula. *Action:* Prevents excessive varus from widening the lateral aspect of the joint. Also helps restrain medial rotation of the tibia. Similar to the MCL, this ligament becomes tight when the knee is extended and slack when the knee is flexed. The LCL, however, is not attached to the lateral meniscus.

Patellar ligament   The patellar ligament is commonly referred to as the patellar tendon. It runs from the distal end of the patella to the tibia. This strong band of tissue is actually the extension of the quadriceps tendon. A portion of this ligament can be used as a donor source of tissue for the repair of other injured structures in the knee, such as the anterior cruciate ligament.

Menisci

The menisci of the knee are crescent-shaped, fibrocartilagenous discs that are attached to the plateau of the tibia. Their function is to act as shock absorbers and distribute the weight of the body evenly through the knee. The wedged menisci also deepen the surface area between the femoral condyles and tibia. This increases the congruency of the two bones and assists with the overall stabilization of the joint. Most of the meniscal tissue does not have a blood supply and therefore relies on movement of the joint to receive its nutrition from the synovial fluid. This lack of vascularization is one reason that meniscal tears do not heal well on their own and often require surgery to excise the torn fragments. Figure 1.2 illustrates the shape and position of the medial and lateral menisci.

Medial meniscus   The medial meniscus is semicircular, or C-shaped, and attaches to the medial portion of the tibial plateau. The meniscus is attached not only to the joint capsule but to the deep portion of the medial collateral ligament as well.

Lateral meniscus   The lateral meniscus is nearly circular, or O-shaped, and attaches to the lateral portion of the tibial plateau. Unlike the medial meniscus, there is no attachment to the lateral collateral ligament, and the lateral meniscus is more mobile.

Bursae

The function of the fluid-filled bursae is to facilitate movement and reduce friction around the bony structures of the knee.

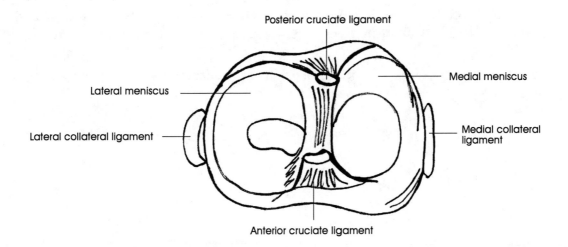

Figure 1.2. Medial and lateral menisci

Suprapatellar (quadriceps) bursa   Located superiorly to the patella, between the femur and the tendon of the quadriceps femoris muscle. This bursa is an extension of the synovial capsule and facilitates normal movement of the quadriceps during full extension and flexion of the knee joint.

Prepatellar bursa   Located superficially between the anterior surface of the patella and the skin. Allows free movement of the skin over the patella when the knee is flexed or extended.

Subcutaneous and deep infrapatellar bursa   The subcutaneous infrapatellar bursa is located between the patellar ligament and the skin. It allows the skin to slide over the tibial tuberosity and to withstand pressure while kneeling in an upright position. The deep infrapatellar bursa is located between the patellar ligament and the anterior surface of the tibia. It allows the patellar ligament to slide over this bony prominence.

Popliteus bursa   Located between the tendon of the popliteus muscle and the lateral tibia. This bursa is an extension of the synovial capsule and allows the popliteus muscle to slide over the tibial condyle.

Pes anserine bursa   Located on the medial surface of the tibia where the pes anserinus inserts. This bursa separates into a number of projections to separate the tendons of the sartorius, gracilis, and the semitendinosus and protects these tendons from the bony prominence.

Gastrocnemius bursa   Located between the medial tendon of the gastrocnemius muscle and the medial femur. This bursa is an extension of the synovial capsule and facilitates normal movement of the gastrocnemius muscle during extension and flexion of the knee joint.

Semimembranosus bursa   Located between the semimembranosus tendon and the medial head of the gastrocnemius muscle.

Study Questions

Complete the following questions. The answer key is on page 107.

1.. True or false: The knee is the largest joint in the body and is classified as a hinge joint.

2. The function of the patellofemoral joint is to _____ the mechanical advantage of the quadriceps muscles and allow _____ force generation across the knee.

3. True or false: A varus alignment of the knee occurs when the distal segment (the tibia) is deviated laterally with respect to the proximal segment (the femur).

4. True or false: The "screw-home mechanism" is an involuntary rotational movement that allows the knee to lock into full extension.

5. The quadriceps consists of the following muscles:

   (1) _____

   (2) _____

   (3) _____

   (4) _____

6. The hamstrings consist of the following muscles:

   (1) _____

   (2) _____

   (3) _____

7. True or false: The gracilis muscle is the longest muscle in the body.

8. Name the four main ligaments in the knee that are essential for providing multidirectional stability to the joint.

   (1) _____

   (2) _____

   (3) _____

   (4) _____

9. True or false: The anterior cruciate ligament prevents excessive backward movement of the tibia on the femur.

10. True or false: The medial collateral ligament prevents excessive valgus from widening the medial aspect of the joint and helps restrain lateral rotation of the tibia.

11. List the eight bursa located around the knee joint:

    (1) _____

    (2) _____

    (3) _____

    (4) _____

    (5) _____

    (6) _____

    (7) _____

    (8) _____

Chapter 2

Dysfunction, Injury, and Rehabilitation

In a normal knee joint all the structures work together smoothly. However, when injury or disease disrupts smooth working of the structures, the result can be knee pain, muscle weakness, and decreased function. The knee joint is one of the most commonly injured areas of the body. Athletes are not the only clients who can experience pain or dysfunction in this joint. The complexity of the joint and its weight-bearing requirements contribute to the many injuries this joint can sustain. In 2003, more than 19.5 million people visited physician's offices due to knee problems (orthoinfo.aaos.org 2009).

Common causes of knee pain and injuries include:

- A blow to the knee from contact sports
- A fall
- Motor vehicle accident
- Repeated stress or overuse
- Sudden turning, pivoting, stopping, cutting from side to side
- Awkward landings from jumping or falling during sports
- Rapidly growing bones
- Degeneration from aging

This chapter describes the disorders and injuries specific to the knee joint and explains the options for surgery and rehabilitation.

Dysfunction

This section describes some of the conditions that can occur in the knee without trauma or injury to the joint. It is important to note that a number of these conditions are frequently seen in younger populations. Clients with these disorders may not be able to participate in vigorous training regimens or certain sports activities. If the client has knee pain, the fitness professional has the responsibility to refer him or her to a qualified medical professional for an evaluation. A physcial therapist will evaluate and attempt to correct any abnormal alignment both above and below the knee to ensure proper knee mechanics. If the client has already been cleared for activity, the fitness professional must properly modify the client's routine so pain is not present during exercise.

Chondromalacia Patella

Chondromalacia patella is the softening and degeneration of the cartilage underneath the kneecap. With this condition, the undersurface of the patella becomes uneven and loses its smoothness. There are two main groups of people who suffer from this condition. One group consists of adults over the age of 50 and the other is teenagers. Chondromalacia patella in older clients may be a sign of arthritis, and the breakdown of cartilage is due to the natural process of aging. Younger clients, however, may have symptoms due to excessive or uneven pressure on the patella.

One common cause of this condition is muscle imbalance resulting in the abnormal alignment of the patella as it slides over the femur during flexion and extension of the knee. Malalignment of the patella, or repeated tracking of the patella along the wrong pathway, increases the pressure on the cartilage under the patella and causes the cartilage to wear down, erode, or fray. In this condition the patella usually tracks to the lateral aspect, or outside, of the femur. The abnormal patellar tracking is also known as patellofemoral syndrome, and it will be discussed in more detail in the next section.

Symptoms of chondromalacia patella include pain that is aggravated with activities such as running, jumping, climbing stairs, and prolonged sitting. Squatting or deep knee bends can cause increased pain, pressure, and effusion around the knee joint. The person may sometimes hear grating, or crepitus, or feel a grinding sensation when flexing and extending his or her knee. This condition is commonly seen in young females, individuals with pronated (flat) feet or "knock-knees," and people who have unusually shaped patellas. Dislocation, fracture, or other injury to the patella can also predispose clients to chondromalacia patella.

Diagnosis is made by a physician's examination, and occasionally by using radiographs (x-rays), magnetic resonance imaging (MRI), or arthroscopy. Arthroscopy is a surgical technique that involves making a few tiny incisions around the knee through which a small camera and other surgical tools are inserted for the purposes of examining and repairing internal knee problems. In severe cases the surgeon may try to treat the fraying cartilage arthroscopically by smoothing out the undersurface of the patella. Before surgery is considered, conservative treatment is commonly prescribed. This involves rest, ice, and nonsteroidal anti-inflammatory drugs for pain and inflammation.

Physical therapy is often indicated to begin a selective strengthening and stretching program for the muscles surrounding the joint. Physical therapy can also employ treatment techniques such as iliotibial band stretching, patellar mobilization, and patellar taping in order to equalize the pull on the patella. The primary goal of treatment is to facilitate the patella to move along the proper pathway during the contraction of the quadriceps. If the patella tracks laterally, exercises to selectively strengthen the inner portion of the quadriceps can assist in bringing the patella into a more centralized position for tracking. Shoe orthotics may also help those clients with pronated (flat) feet. Another option is bracing the knee when engaged in sports or other activities in order to improve the alignment of the patella.

Patellofemoral Syndrome

Patellofemoral syndrome occurs when the patella does not glide evenly on the femur or is not properly aligned in the patellofemoral groove. The cause of the patellar malalignment may include muscle imbalance around the knee joint, abnormal rotation of the hip or tibia, or an altered angle between the femur and the tibia. Abnormalities of the foot and ankle, such as pronated feet, may also contribute to the problem. Adolescents and young females are affected most frequently.

As mentioned previously, patellofemoral syndrome is also commonly referred to as chondromalacia patella. The names are used interchangeably because the malalignment of the patella typically leads to the wearing down of the patellar cartilage, or chondromalacia patella. Nevertheless, these conditions are not the same, and one disorder does not have to be present for the other condition to occur. For instance, chondromalacia patella may occur with the natural aging process, but the client may not exhibit altered alignment of the patella. Similarly, a client may have a patella alignment problem that has not yet caused the patellar cartilage to wear down.

Although the probable causes of patellofemoral syndrome will be discussed separately, it is likely that the etiology, or cause, of the syndrome is multifactorial in nature.

Muscle imbalance or weakness around the knee   Various forces are responsible for the movement of the patella; however, the quadriceps muscle group is the main stabilizer of the patellofemoral joint. The vastus medialis muscle pulls the patella medially, or toward the inside of the knee, while the vastus lateralis muscle counteracts this force by pulling it laterally. The rectus femoris and vastus intermedius muscles stabilize the patella centrally. If one of these muscles is stronger than the others, the patella is pulled, or tracks, preferentially to one side. Likewise, if one of the quadricep muscles is weak, the other muscles can overpower it and cause the patella to track preferentially to one side. The abnormal tracking can be the cause of knee pain and degeneration of the cartilage under the patella. In most cases the patella tracks too far laterally due to vastus medialis weakness or imbalance between the relative strengths of the vastus medialis and the vastus lateralis. Another contribution to lateral tracking is tightness of the iliotibial band, which is a dense group of fibrous connective tissue on the outside of the leg.

In addition, if the quadricep muscles are weak, pain can result from the extra pressure between the patella and the femur during knee flexion. Activities such as running, climbing, descending stairs, and even prolonged sitting can exacerbate the pain symptoms if the muscles are not strong enough to support the joint. Tightness or inflexibility of the hamstring muscles can place more posterior force on the knee, causing the pressure to increase between the patella and femur.

Muscles surrounding the hip, including the abductors and lateral rotators, can also contribute to knee instability and pain. The hip abductors, primarily the gluteus medius, gluteus minimus, and tensor fascia latae, as well as the lateral rotators, act eccentrically to control forces at the knee. If these muscles are weak, they can allow increased femoral medial rotation and valgus knee movements. This in turn can place excessive compressive force on the patellofemoral joint and lead to patellofemoral syndrome.

Foot abnormalities and rotation of the hip or tibia   Another possible cause of patellofemoral syndrome is the position of the foot in standing. If the client has flat (pronated) feet, the medial arch lacks support, which causes a compensatory rotation of the tibia and femur. This rotation causes increased stress at the knee and disrupts the normal alignment of the patella. Furthermore, a tight or inflexible gastrocnemius muscle can lead to compensatory foot pronation as well. Arch supports or custom-made orthotics oftentimes can alleviate this problem. Likewise, a client with a high-arched foot also has compensatory rotation at the tibia and femur, along with decreased cushioning for the leg when the foot hits the ground. This in turn places more stress on the knee and patellofemoral joint, especially with high-impact activities such as running. Orthotics, arch supports, and proper footwear can provide the proper support needed at the foot in order to decrease or alleviate the knee pain.

Altered angle between the femur and the tibia (Q-angle)   The Q-angle, or quadriceps angle, is the angle between a line connecting the anterior superior iliac spine of the pelvis to the midpoint of the patella and the extension of a line connecting the tibia tubercle and the midpoint of the patella. Figures 2.1 and 2.2 illustrate how the Q-angle of the knee is measured. The line between the pelvis and the midpoint of the patella is an estimate of the line of pull of the quadriceps muscle. A Q-angle greater than 20 degrees is considered abnormal and indicates an excessive lateral force on the patella, which may

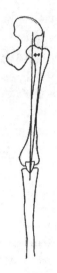

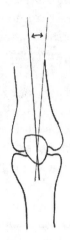

Figure 2.1. Measurement of the Q-angle   Figure 2.2. Q-angle

predispose it to pathologic changes. Females typically have larger Q-angles than men due to the wider pelvis. Studies have shown that Q-angles vary greatly between individuals. Subjects with "normal" Q-angles may present with severe knee pain, while those with larger angles may not have any symptoms. Therefore, caution should be used when looking at the Q-angle as a diagnostic tool or predictor of clients with knee pain.

Symptoms of patellofemoral syndrome include pain underneath or around the patella that increases with weight-bearing activities or prolonged sitting. Diagnosis is based on a physician's examination and the client's history of symptoms. Radiographs may be ordered to rule out other conditions. Initial treatment consists of rest, ice, nonsteroidal anti-inflammatories, and activity modification. A client whose symptoms occur with sitting can benefit from straightening out the leg, walking periodically, or changing positions as needed.

Physical therapy is often recommended for specific muscle strengthening exercises and flexibility training for the iliotibial band, hamstring, and gastrocnemius muscles. As with chondromalacia patella, the primary goal of treatment is to facilitate the patella to move along the proper pathway during quadriceps contraction. If the patella tracks laterally, exercises to selectively strengthen the vastus medialis can assist in bringing the patella into a more centralized position during knee flexion and extension.

Knee braces with a hole cut out for the patella are often used to help keep the patella from deviating laterally, thereby decreasing knee pain. There is a lack of consensus in the literature regarding the efficacy of these braces due to the absence of well-controlled studies. Nevertheless, those who wear the patellofemoral braces have reported significant subjective improvements in pain and disability. Knee braces may be beneficial in controlling the symptoms while engaged in sporting activities, but they should not be worn at all times because continuous use can lead to weakening of the quadriceps muscle and further exacerbate patellofemoral issues. In general, the use of patellofemoral braces is no substitute for a well-designed exercise program for strengthening muscles and increasing flexibility of the knee.

Surgery is usually considered to be the last treatment option for patellofemoral syndrome. The surgical technique to correct this condition is called a lateral retinacular release. The retinaculum is fibrous tissue located on either side of the patella that helps keep the patella centrally aligned. The lateral retinaculum has fibers that run to the iliotibial band and the vastus lateralis. If these fibers are contributing to the lateral misalignment of the patella, they are cut during the surgery, and the kneecap is able to return to a more centralized position. Rehabilitation is usually initiated after surgery to retrain and strengthen the muscles around the knee.

Popliteal (Baker's) Cysts

Popliteal, or Baker's, cysts are characterized by visible swelling on the posterior aspect of the knee, which is caused by an accumulation of synovial fluid escaping from the knee joint capsule. The cyst may or may not be tender and may or may not interfere with flexion or extension of the knee. A popliteal cyst may be a symptom of another underlying problem in the knee, such as a meniscal tear or osteoarthritis. Diagnosis can be made by a doctor's examination or radiograph. Treatment options include aspiration or removal of the fluid by needle, anti-inflammatory medications, cortisone injections, and physical therapy.

Osgood-Schlatter Disease

Osgood-Schlatter disease occurs when the patellar ligament pulls away from its insertion on the tibial tuberosity. It is seen more frequently in an active population of children who are involved in running and jumping activities. Frequent stair climbing or deep knee bending can also worsen the symptoms. Sports that may contribute to this condition include football, soccer, basketball, gymnastics, and ballet. In addition, adolescent boys ages 10 to 16 who are having a growth spurt can also be affected.

Frequent pulling of the ligament at the insertion site causes the bone to harden, and a lump can sometimes be felt over the tibial tuberosity. Other symptoms include pain, inflammation, and swelling on the front of the tibia. A radiograph is typically used to diagnose Osgood-Schlatter disease, along with an examination by a physician. Treatment consists of rest, nonsteroidal anti-inflammatories, pain medication, and ice. Weight-bearing activities can aggravate the condition and increase pain. Oftentimes, the bone will heal as the child grows, and the condition will resolve itself. Children may be instructed to stop their sports activities for two to four months so healing can occur. Physical therapy may be indicated for pain control and to prescribe exercises for gentle strengthening. The child can gradually return to sporting activity as the pain and inflammation decrease.

Osteochondritis Dissecans

Osteochondritis dissecans occurs when a small piece of cartilage or bone becomes separated from the condyle of the femur. The fragment may stay in place or fall into the joint space, causing pain and instability of the knee joint. This condition may be the result of a repetitive force injury to the bone that causes a loss of blood supply to that area. Symptoms may include pain and swelling in the joint, a catching or locking sensation with movement, and stiffness after rest. Although this condition is typically seen in active, younger children, adults can also be affected. Sports like tennis, basketball, and gymnastics that involve jumping, cutting, and pivoting can place individuals at risk. Diagnosis can usually be made by radiographs, but other tests, such as an MRI or computerized tomography (CT) scan, may also be ordered to determine the full extent of the damage and rule out any other problems within the knee. Treatment includes rest, immobilization, nonsteroidal anti-inflammatories, and physical therapy for stretching, ROM, and gentle strengthening.

Juvenile osteochondritis dissecans has a better chance of healing itself because the bones are still maturing and growing. Nonsurgical treatment may take 10 to 18 months. Surgery may be necessary to remove the loose body from the joint space, or the surgeon may try to reattach the bone fragment or place a graft where the lesion is located. With damage to the surface of the joint, degenerative osteoarthritis can develop later due to the increased wear and tear on the joint.

Iliotibial Band Syndrome

Iliotibial band syndrome (ITBS) is the result of chronic irritation and inflammation of a dense group of fibrous connective tissue known as the iliotibial band (ITB). This band of fascia runs from the gluteus maximus and tensor fascia latae muscles down to the lateral condyle of the femur and the lateral portion of the tibia. The function of the iliotibial band is to assist with hip abduction—moving the leg away from the body. During ambulation or running, however, the iliotibial band controls or decelerates adduction of the leg that occurs when the foot hits the ground. Irritation of the ITB is caused by overuse, or repetitive flexion and extension of the knee. As the knee is flexed and extended, the insertion of the band repetitively rubs over the condyle of the femur, leading to irritation. Running, hiking, and vigorous walking can all contribute to the tension on the ITB. Studies indicate that 4.3% to 7.5% of long-distance runners experience iliotibial band syndrome (Martinez, Honsik, and Lorenzo 2006). Cyclists may also experience ITBS if the position of the bike seat is too high. Increased varus at the knee or pronation of the foot can also predispose an athlete to iliotibial band syndrome.

The most common symptom of ITBS is pain along the outside of the knee or lateral leg, which increases during physical activity. The client may also complain of pain when walking up or down stairs, running hills, or during heel strike (when the foot hits the ground). Initial treatment of this condition includes rest, ice, and nonsteroidal anti-inflammatories. Heat and stretching can then be used prior to activity. Physical therapy may be recommended to initiate a stretching program, help the person modify his or her training routine, or evaluate the person's foot biomechanics for orthotics. After the pain and inflammation have been reduced, strengthening can be initiated with a gradual return to activity.

Arthritis

It is estimated that approximately 27 million Americans suffer from osteoarthritis (Arthritis Foundation 2009). Osteoarthritis is a degenerative joint disease that causes destruction of a joint, resulting in pain and impaired movement. Diagnosis is primarily made through radiographs. Symptoms include pain or stiffness in the joint, limitations in joint movement, and swelling. Although there is no definitive cause of arthritis, researchers believe that there are a number of risk factors for the disease, which include joint stress, previous injury, the aging process, and being overweight. Osteoarthritis is commonly treated with nonsteroidal anti-inflammatories and other conservative measures. Exercise for strengthening the muscles around the joint helps to increase the joint's stability while decreasing the friction between the joint surfaces. Physical therapy must address the overall alignment both above and below the knee joint when treating clients with arthritis in order to decrease the abnormal mechanics and compressive forces on the joint. Surgery to replace the knee joint is also an option for those with severe pain that interferes with everyday activities. According to the American Academy of Orthopaedic Surgeons (AAOS), approximately 581,000 total knee replacement surgeries are performed each year (AAOS 2009). Those who undergo total knee replacement, or total knee arthroplasty, have a chance to live pain free and resume normal activities of daily living. The fitness professional can play an invaluable role in encouraging symmetrical knee flexibility and strength to help the client make the most of his or her postsurgical knee and avoid another knee replacement or revision.

Injury

Injury to the knee joint is common. The muscles, ligaments, and other supporting structures in and around the knee can easily be disrupted or damaged while engaged in sports activities or even simple activities of daily living. The severity of an injury can range from minor (a mild sprain or stretch of the ligament) to severe (a complete tear or rupture). In addition, people may injure more than one structure in a single traumatic event.

Athletes are commonly affected by injuries to the knee. In a survey conducted of high school athletes, the knee was the second most frequently injured body site overall, with boys' football and wrestling and girls' soccer and basketball recording the highest rates of knee injury (Ingram et al. 2008). The most common knee injuries according to this study were incomplete ligament tears, contusions, complete ligament tears, torn menisci, fractures/dislocations, and muscle tears. Interestingly, researchers also found that while boys had a higher overall rate of knee injury, girls' knee injuries were more severe. Girls were also found to be twice as likely to experience major knee injuries as a result of noncontact mechanisms, often involving landing, jumping, and pivoting (Ingram et al. 2008).

This section gives a description of common knee injuries. It is imperative that a client who complains of knee pain be given a thorough evaluation by a medical professional or physical therapist before initiating an exercise routine. Many injuries can become worse if too much strain is placed on the knee or the client is given improper exercises. Fortunately, performing a proper strength training and stability exercise routine may also help reduce the chance of injury.

It is important to remember that every client and every injury should be treated individually. The information provided is intended to give the fitness professional a basic idea of the rehabilitation and treatment that is involved with these types of conditions. Always remember to seek counsel from a physician or physical therapist when working with a client who has had a recent knee injury.

Strains and Sprains

Strains are caused by overstretching a muscle or tendon. A sprain occurs when a ligament is injured. The mechanism of injury could be a fall, a direct blow to the knee joint, or the result of repetitive activities such as bending and lifting. Pain, irritation, and swelling in the area of injury are some common symptoms. Typical rehabilitation consists of ice, rest, possible immobilization with a knee brace, nonsteroidal anti-inflammatories, muscle relaxants or pain medication, and then heat with stretching. After this initial period of rest and pain reduction, strengthening can be initiated in order to counteract any muscle weakness caused by inactivity. Gradual return to activity is allowed once the strengthening exercises can be performed without discomfort.

Tendonitis

Tendonitis is an inflammation of the tendon resulting from overuse, trauma, or excessive tensile forces on the tendon. Patellar tendonitis is also known as "jumper's knee" because the repetitive strain of jumping may increase the irritation to the tendon. Ice, rest, and the use of nonsteroidal anti-inflammatories are all indicated for early treatment of tendonitis. Management of this condition by a physician or physical therapist focuses on reducing the pain and inflammation. Physical therapy may also use modalities such as ultrasound, electrical stimulation, ice, and stretching exercises. Strengthening exercises can then be incorporated into an exercise program in order to return the individual to daily or recreational activities.

Bursitis

Bursitis is an inflammation of the bursa usually caused by overuse or trauma. Prepatellar bursitis is one common form of bursitis caused by friction between the skin and the patella. This condition is seen in people who work on their knees without using kneepads, such as roofers, carpet layers, and floor tilers.

Initial management of bursitis calls for reducing the pain and inflammation before restoring functional activities. Physical therapy may also be initiated with a physician's referral. Treatment for bursitis is similar to tendonitis and involves the use of the same modalities with a gradual return to activities.

Occasionally a client may report that he or she is experiencing a flare-up of tendonitis or bursitis. Encourage your client to see a physician before starting an exercise routine. Continued activity will further inflame the structures and lead to increased pain and dysfunction. If the client has already been evaluated by a physician or physical therapist, the best option is to postpone any training until the symptoms have completely resolved.

Ligament Tears

Ligament tears of the knee are frequently associated with sports injuries. Tears are typically graded according to their severity.

Grade I   Mild tear, no gross loss of integrity of ligament fibers. No hypermobility or gross instability of joint.

Grade II   Moderate (partial) tear, partial loss of integrity of ligament fibers. Mild instability of joint.

Grade III   Severe tear or complete rupture of the ligament. Moderate to severe hypermobility of joint.

In general, Grade I and Grade II ligament injuries do not require surgery and can be treated with a rehabilitation program to manage pain, increase range of motion, decrease swelling, and gradually increase strength. Following a mild to moderate knee ligament injury, the client should be able to return to a normal level of activity. With physician approval, fitness professionals may be able to start working with these types of clients to help regain their strength and improve the stability of their knee. Grade III tears often require surgical intervention followed by intensive physical rehabilitation.

Anterior Cruciate Ligament (ACL) Tear

Each year approximately 80,000 to 250,000 ACL injuries occur (Griffin et al. 2006). Many of these injuries occur in young athletes 15 to 25 years of age. A tear occurs when the ACL is unable to restrain anterior translation of the tibia on the femur or when a force against the anterior thigh drives the femur backward on the tibia when the knee is close to full extension. An anterior cruciate ligament tear can potentially cost an athlete an entire season away from his or her sport. In addition, approximately 50% of clients with ACL injuries also have meniscal tears (Hubbell and Schwartz 2006).

The anterior cruciate ligament can potentially be injured in several ways during functional or recreational activities, such as:

- Changing direction rapidly
- Stopping suddenly
- Landing from a jump
- Direct contact or collision

Injuries to the ACL are most often a result of low-velocity, noncontact deceleration motions or contact injuries with a rotational component. Twisting, hyperextension, or valgus stress to the knee may also be hazardous to the ACL and cause injury during sports activities. At the time of the ACL injury, the position of the leg often "displays tibial rotation, apparent knee valgus, foot pronation, and a relatively extended knee and hip" (Griffin et al. 2006, 1521).

An individual who sustains an injury to the ACL will often feel or hear an audible pop that occurs when changing direction, cutting, or landing from a jump (usually with a combination of hyperextension and pivoting). Edema will develop quickly and the individual will experience an increase in pain with difficulty bearing weight on the affected leg. A physician's examination and an MRI will confirm the diagnosis. Ice, rest, immobilization, and physical therapy may be ordered for initial management of the injury. The overall goal of conservative treatment is to gain full range of motion and strength of the knee. Nonoperative treatment may be considered for the elderly population or for athletes who do not participate in sports that involve pivoting, cutting, or quick deceleration movements, such as cycling or swimming.

Without surgical intervention the knee is at an even greater risk for degenerative wear and tear secondary to the decreased stability once provided by the ACL. The menisci are also predisposed to injury due to the additional forces that can potentially damage and abrade the cartilage. Furthermore, the other stabilizing ligaments will be stressed as they attempt to compensate for the decreased stability of the knee; specifically, the MCL, which becomes the primary restraint to anterior tibial translation when the ACL is injured.

When deciding on surgery, the physician will consider the following factors:

- Preinjury activity level (sedentary versus athlete)
- Desire to return to high-demand sports (e.g., basketball, football, soccer)
- Associated injuries (medial collateral ligament tear or meniscal tear)
- Severity of laxity
- Patient expectations

The Centers for Disease Control and Prevention (CDC) has estimated that approximately 100,000 ACL reconstructions are performed annually (Griffin et al. 2006). There are a number of techniques used to reconstruct the ACL arthroscopically. Each technique has its own associated benefits and drawbacks and will be chosen according to the surgeon's preference. Three of the surgical techniques will be described briefly.

Patellar tendon autograft (bone-tendon-bone graft)   With the patellar tendon graft, the central portion of the patellar tendon is removed along with a small piece of bone from both the patella and the tibia at each end of the tendon. The bone on each end allows for the graft to be securely fixed with screws inside the tunnels that are drilled in the femur and tibia. The tunnels are located very close to the position of the original ACL attachments. As healing occurs, the tunnels in the bone fill in to further secure the graft tendon in place. This technique was the first successful graft to be used in modern ACL surgery and is considered to be the "gold standard" for ACL reconstruction. Athletes are usually able to return to their preinjury sport after rehabilitation is complete. Drawbacks of using this technique include a higher incidence of anterior knee pain and inflammation of the patellar tendon, possibly leading to patellar tendonitis.

Hamstring tendon autograft   The hamstring tendon autograft involves the removal of a portion of the semitendinosus or gracilis tendons, which are then used to replace the ACL. Special screws are used to fix the tendon within the bone tunnel. This graft technique is associated with less anterior knee pain and is easier to harvest than the patellar tendon. One drawback is the fixation, which does not have bone to anchor it. Some also believe that this technique is more susceptible to elongation of the graft itself. Most athletes do not notice a decrease in agility or strength of the hamstrings with this type of technique.

Allograft transfer   Allografts are tissue taken from a cadaver. The proposed advantages include decreased surgical time, sparing the individual's own tissue, and reducing potential donor-site complications. Nevertheless, allografts are associated with a risk of viral transmission and infection. Allografts may also be used for revisions if another ACL reconstruction technique has failed.

Postsurgery Physical Therapy

Physical therapy is essential for the rehabilitation of the knee after ACL reconstruction. Most therapy protocols will divide the rehabilitation into phases. The first phase concentrates on reducing pain, decreasing edema, increasing quadriceps control, and achieving increased range of motion. The second phase involves the maintenance of full range of motion and improving the strength of the quadriceps and hamstrings. The final phase is focused on dynamic and sport-specific exercises in order to return higher-level clients to their preinjury sports participation. Rehabilitation following ACL reconstruction is lengthy. An athlete with this type of injury may require up to a year before returning to full sports activity without restrictions. Overall, the long-term success rate for ACL reconstruction is 82% to 95% (Hubbell and Schwartz 2006). Nevertheless, clients are still at risk for posttraumatic osteoarthritis and future meniscal injury following ACL injury and subsequent surgery. The fitness professional can play a role in a client's long-term, successful outcome by designing a program of strengthening exercises to improve the overall stability of the knee.

Functional Braces

Much debate has centered on the use of functional braces after ACL reconstruction to help increase the stability of the knee and prevent further injury when involved in sports activities. Wearing a knee brace is thought to decrease the stress on the ACL; however, studies have shown that functional bracing can only limit the anterior translation of the tibia on the femur at lower loads. In fact, a recent study by Birmingham et al. in 2008 does not support the recommendation of using a functional knee brace after reconstruction of the ACL. Their research showed that functional knee braces were no better than neoprene sleeves at protecting the knee following ACL surgery. In a related study, reviewers of 12 separate randomized, controlled trials found "no evidence that pain, range of motion, graft stability, or protection from subsequent injury were affected by brace use..." (Wright and Fetzer 2007, 162). Nevertheless, the decision whether to use a functional brace after an ACL reconstruction surgery is left to the surgeon's discretion.

Causative Factors in ACL Injuries

When matched for activities, females have a greater prevalence for ACL injury than males. Most noncontact injuries occur during landing from a jump, decelerating, or pivoting during running. The incidence of noncontact ACL injuries remains greater in sports such as soccer, basketball, volleyball, and gymnastics that require rapid deceleration during cutting, pivoting, landing, and change in directions. The literature reveals that the rate of injury is anywhere from 2 to 10 times greater for females. It has been hypothesized that some of these differences may be due to limb alignment and anatomic differences, sex hormones and joint laxity, different strength-to-weight ratios, alterations in muscle activation, movement, and recruitment patterns, as well as differences in training. However, further studies are needed to determine any definitive causes. Some of the theories are discussed below.

ACL Injury Rate among Females

Anatomic differences are thought to play a role in the difference of ACL injury rate between males and females. The notch between the condyles of the femur where the ACL passes through is narrower in females than in males. Therefore, the ACL is more susceptible to getting pinched as the knee flexes and extends, which can lead to a tear or rupture of the ligament. A greater Q-angle at the knee may also place more strain on the ligament. As mentioned previously, the Q-angle is the angle at which the femur meets the tibia and it is usually larger in women due to a wider pelvis. The larger the angle, the greater the stress placed on the knee.

Another theory explaining the difference in injury rates between males and females is the possible effect of female sex hormones on the ACL structure. Research has shown that a greater number of injuries occur in the follicular phase of the menstrual cycle. Although the evidence is not conclusive, hormones may play a role in ligamentous laxity and joint stability, which may affect the rate of ACL injury.

Alterations in movement patterns and muscle activation have also been studied as a possible way of explaining the discrepancy between male and female injury rates. For example, research has shown that in comparison to men, women "appear to land a jump, cut, and pivot with less knee and hip flexion, increased knee valgus, increased internal rotation of the hip, increased external rotation of the tibia, less knee joint stiffness, and high quadriceps activity relative to hamstring activity" (Griffin et al. 2006, 1519). In fact, studies have shown that one of the common factors involved in noncontact ACL ruptures is the lower extremity in a position of valgus. One study found that female subjects landed with significantly greater knee valgus than did the male subjects (Ford et al. 2003). As mentioned previously, the valgus position of the lower extremity has been viewed as a perilous position for the knee. To further illustrate this, Hewett et al. in 2005 found that dynamic knee valgus measures during a jump-landing task were predictive of future ACL risk in females that were participating in a high-risk sport, such as basketball, soccer, and volleyball.

Muscle strength and activation may also be contributing factors to the higher ACL injury rate seen among females. Compared with males, females have reduced muscle strength in proportion to bone size. It is speculated that women may rely more on the ACL to hold the knee in place than on the muscles, and if the ACL is continually stressed, the ligament may be more prone to rupture. In addition, females have been shown to have greater activation of the quadriceps over the hamstring muscles. Studies demonstrate that "female athletes contract their quadriceps to a much greater degree than the hamstrings compared with male athletes at landing and in response to an anterior tibial translation" (Hewett 2000, 316). The hamstrings are considered to be ACL agonists, meaning they help resist forces that strain the ACL. Furthermore, the hamstrings are thought to increase the stability of the knee by resisting the anterior shear forces on the tibia and functioning as a joint compressor. The quadriceps, however, are ACL antagonists and can significantly increase the strain on the ACL during a muscle contraction with the knee in flexion. In 1996, Hewett et al. demonstrated that with training, female high school athletes could correct their hamstring strength imbalances and increase their hamstring power. This study went on to say that the same training program could decrease the landing forces in the knee, thereby potentially decreasing the number of injuries that occur when female athletes land from a jump.

ACL Injury Prevention

Although it is not definitively known what causes women to be more prone to ACL injury, it has been shown in scientific studies that a neuromuscular training program can lower the risk of ACL injury in female athletes. Evidence suggests that exercise-based ACL prevention programs may alter key risk factors in ACL injury. In 1999, Hewett et al. showed that a neuromuscular training program could decrease the incidence of serious knee injury in female athletes by three to four times. A neuromuscular training program that improves strength and flexibility and teaches athletes correct jumping and landing techniques may help to prevent excessive stress on the ACL. Even if differences in strength, flexibility, and training account for only a small percentage of the female injury rate, it would have a tremendous effect on the number of overall knee injuries.

Successful neuromuscular training programs appear to include one or several of the following components: traditional stretching and strengthening activities, aerobic conditioning, agilities, plyometrics, and risk awareness training. Plyometric exercises in particular have been found to "decrease landing forces, decrease varus/valgus moments, and increase effective muscle activation" (Griffin et al. 2006, 1522).

One program in particular has had a significant effect on lowering the risk of ACL injuries in female soccer players. The program was developed by a team of physicians, physical therapists, athletic trainers, and coaches at the Santa Monica Orthopaedic and Sports Medicine Foundation. The Prevent injury, Enhance Performance (PEP) program is a highly specific 15-minute training session that takes the place of a traditional warm-up (The Santa Monica Orthopedic and Sports Medicine Group 2009). The goals of the program are to:

- Avoid vulnerable positions
- Increase flexibility

- Increase strength
- Include plyometric exercises in the training program
- Increase proprioception through agilities

See the appendix for more PEP information.

The program emphasizes proper landing technique when jumping: "stressing 'soft landing' and deep hip and knee flexion as opposed to landing with a 'flat foot' in lower extremity extension" (Mandelbaum et al. 2005, 2). It is recommended that athletes perform this program three times a week during the season. The ultimate goal of the program is to decrease the number of ACL injuries in the female athlete.

A study performed in 2005 by Mandelbaum et al. demonstrated that the PEP program was effective in decreasing the incidence of ACL ligament injuries in a population of female soccer players ages 14 to 18 years. During the first year of the study there was an 88% decrease in ACL injury in the enrolled participants compared with the control group, while in the second year there was a 74% reduction in injury. Although this study looked specifically at female soccer players, the authors state that the results of their study "indicate that a neuromuscular training program, such as the PEP program, may significantly reduce the incidence of severe ACL injuries in the female athlete" (Mandelbaum et al. 2005, 6). Furthermore, the "results of this study were akin to those prevention programs developed for basketball players, amateur and professional soccer players, skiers, and volleyball athletes" (Mandelbaum et al. 2005, 6). According to Holly Silvers, P.T., one of the coauthors of the study, preliminary data showed that the results can be extrapolated for both male and female athletes over the age of 9 participating in court- and field-based sports.

A follow-up study in 2008 by Gilchrist et al. also demonstrated that the incidence of ACL injury in collegiate female soccer players could be reduced with participation in the PEP program. NCAA Division One women's soccer teams were randomly assigned to a control group or intervention group that performed the PEP program three times per week during the season. The results of the study showed that the noncontact ACL injury rate among the intervention participants was 3.3 times lower than in the control group. Furthermore, athletes within the intervention groups who had a history of ACL injury were significantly less likely to suffer another ACL injury while participating in the PEP program.

The PEP program consists of a warm-up, stretching, strengthening, plyometrics, and sport-specific agilities to address potential deficits in the strength and coordination of the stabilizing muscles around the knee joint. According to the program, it is important to use proper technique during all of the exercises. The coaches and trainers need to emphasize correct posture, instruct the execution of straight up-and-down jumps without excessive side-to-side movement, and reinforce soft landings.

Posterior Cruciate Ligament (PCL) Tear

Posterior cruciate ligament tears are less common than anterior cruciate ligament injuries. Injury to this ligament often goes unrecognized. The PCL is injured when the tibia is forced backward in relation to the femur. One mechanism of injury occurs when an individual hits his or her knees on the dashboard in a motor vehicle accident. Another example is a football player falling on a bent knee. Hyperextension of the knee and excessive rotation may also be responsible for PCL tears. A knee with an isolated PCL tear is less likely to show gross instability of the knee when examined.

Typical symptoms of a posterior cruciate ligament injury include pain with swelling that occurs quickly after the injury, difficulty walking, and feeling as though the knee may give out. Diagnosis is made with a physician's evaluation and an MRI. Initial treatment includes ice, rest, immobilization, and physical therapy. Physical therapy in nonoperative cases consists of increasing weight bearing, improving range of motion, and increasing knee strength. After a few months, advanced strengthening exercises and sport-specific training can be initiated and progressed as tolerated.

It is possible for a partial PCL tear to heal enough on its own so that an athlete can return to sports without knee stability problems. One long-term follow-up study following nonoperative treatment for PCL injuries revealed that after completing a rehabilitation program, 68% of the patients returned to their previous level of competitive function; however, 44% developed significant degenerative changes and 31% showed radiographic signs of arthritis (Parolie and Bergfeld 1986). Nevertheless, surgery is usually recommended if the ligament has been completely torn with resulting gross instability of the knee or there are other injuries present.

Controversy exists in the literature regarding the treatment of PCL injuries. Recommendations support both operative and nonoperative treatments. PCL reconstruction requires careful attention to detail and precise surgical technique due to the delicate nerves and blood vessels that run along the back of the knee. Similar to ACL reconstruction, the grafts for the PCL are taken from the patellar tendon or the hamstrings and are held in place by screws within the tunnels that are drilled into the femur and tibia. The tunnels are aligned with the original attachments of the PCL.

Physical therapy following this surgery is similar to the phases of rehabilitation for ACL reconstruction. Stretching for improved range of motion, strengthening exercises, and modalities for pain and swelling are indicated initially. After a few months, the goals of rehabilitation are focused on increasing strength, power, and endurance. Functional strengthening and sport-specific training is later incorporated and advanced as tolerated. Full recovery typically requires 6 to 12 months but may be slower if other injuries are present.

Medial Collateral Ligament (MCL) Tear

The medial collateral ligament is one of the most commonly injured knee ligaments; however, the incidence of MCL injuries is difficult to determine because of the wide range in severity. Some injuries to the MCL are so minor that they may never be evaluated by a physician or physical therapist. Oftentimes the ACL and the medial meniscus are also injured with the MCL. When comparing the tensile strength of the ligaments in the knee, the MCL is twice as strong as the ACL, and the ACL appears to have slightly less strength than the PCL.

The medial collateral ligament may be injured in both contact and noncontact sports. Contact injuries involve a direct load to the outside of the leg that forces the knee into a valgus position. These types of injuries are usually responsible for a complete tear of the ligament. One common mechanism of injury is the "clip" block in football when a player is tackled from the side. Noncontact, or indirect, injuries are seen with movements such as cutting, pivoting, and quick deceleration. These movements are more likely to cause partial tears or sprains.

Symptoms of an MCL tear include pain over the inside of the knee joint, swelling, stiffness, and difficulty bearing weight on the affected leg. Definitive diagnosis is made through a physician's examination and an MRI. Ligament tears are initially treated with rest, nonsteroidal anti-inflammatories, protective weight bearing with crutches, and the possible use of a knee splint or brace. Physical therapy treatment is focused on restoring range of motion, decreasing pain and swelling, and regaining strength. Advanced rehabilitation involves the use of sport-specific exercises and drills to return the athlete to preinjury level. Return to sport is allowed when agility testing can be performed without pain. Depending on the severity of the tear, it may take three to nine months before the athlete is able to return to full preinjury activities. Surgical intervention is rarely required unless there is another associated injury, such as an ACL tear.

Lateral Collateral Ligament (LCL) Tear

The lateral collateral ligament is injured when a force is directed at the inside of the leg and forces the knee into a varus position. The LCL is less commonly injured than the MCL because the opposite leg usually blocks against direct blows to the medial aspect of the knee. Nevertheless, the knee is vulnerable to this type of hit whenever the leg is extended in front of the body, such as when attempting to kick a soccer ball or when lunging forward to make a tackle.

Symptoms of an LCL tear include pain over the outside of the knee joint, swelling, stiffness, and difficulty bearing weight on the affected leg. Definitive diagnosis is made through a physician's examination and an MRI. LCL tears are treated similarly to an injury of the MCL, with ice, nonsteroidal anti-inflammatories, protective weight bearing, and a knee splint prescribed initially. The goals of rehabilitation are also similar. Athletes

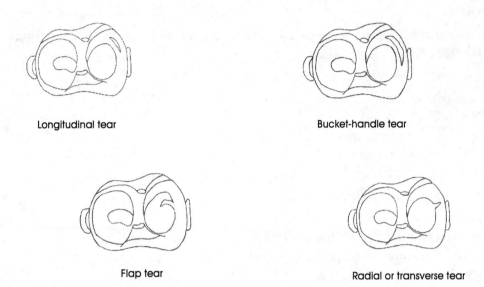

Figure 2.3. Meniscal tears

may return to sports when they regain full strength and ROM and when they are free of pain with functional activities and sport-related drills. Surgical intervention is not usually recommended unless there is concomitant damage to other ligaments or the posterolateral capsule complex.

Meniscal Tears

Meniscal tears are a common condition that can occur during any type of activity. They often occur in conjunction with a torn ligament. The "terrible triad" refers to a simultaneous injury of three structures in the knee: the anterior cruciate ligament, the medial collateral ligament, and the medial meniscus.

The following are examples of meniscal tears:

Degenerative tear   The edges of the menisci become frayed or jagged due to wear and tear of the joint.

Longitudinal tear   Runs along the length of the meniscus.

Bucket-handle tear   Similar to a longitudinal tear; however, a portion of the meniscus becomes detached and forms a flap that resembles a bucket handle.

Flap tear   Also similar to a longitudinal tear but with a small segment of the fragmented meniscus displaced.

Radial or transverse tear   Extends from the outer edge of the meniscus or perpendicular to the free edge of the meniscus.

The symptoms of a meniscal tear are:

- History of trauma or twisting of the knee
- Pain along the joint line of the knee
- Swelling of the knee within 24–48 hours of the injury
- Difficulty bending or extending the knee fully
- Clicking, popping, or locking when attempting to move the knee

It is not unusual for a client to have a meniscal injury and be unable to recall a specific incident that caused the damage to the cartilage.

Diagnosis of a meniscal tear is made through an MRI. Conservative treatment includes ice, rest, knee bracing, nonsteroidal anti-inflammatories, and physical therapy. The goals of physical therapy are to minimize swelling, normalize pain-free range of motion, prevent atrophy of the muscles, and return the individual to activities of daily living and recreation.

Arthroscopic surgery may be necessary to repair the tear. Left untreated, the tear may increase in size and cause abrasion of the cartilage, resulting in arthritis. Approximately 850,000 meniscal surgeries are performed each year (Baker and Lubowitz 2008). The goal of surgery is to preserve as much of the meniscal cartilage as possible. Partial meniscectomy, or removal of the torn meniscus, is the surgical technique performed on the portion of the meniscus that is unable to be repaired. The torn tissue is resected, or removed, and the remaining healthy tissue is contoured and smoothed to become a more stable and balanced surface.

Meniscal repair, or suturing the torn piece back in place, may be performed if the tear is located where the blood supply is more prevalent and the chances of healing are greater. Smoothing and abrading the torn edges and borders of the meniscus may also be performed with this surgical repair technique. Studies have shown that resection of 15% to 34% of a meniscus may increase contact pressure (on the knee) by more than 350% (Baker and Lubowitz 2008). Furthermore, normal knees have 20% better shock-absorbing capacity than knees that have undergone a meniscectomy (Baker and Lubowitz 2008).

Physical therapy is typically prescribed after surgery for muscle strengthening and pain control. Some surgeons may restrict weight bearing on the affected leg for a few weeks to allow for healing. Goals in physical therapy include decreasing pain, restoring full range of motion and strength in the knee, and the eventual return to sports activity. Return to play depends on the extent of the injury, the person's age and activity level, as well as the presence of other associated injuries, such as a ligament tear.

Medial meniscus tear.   The medial meniscus is torn more frequently than the lateral meniscus because of its decreased mobility, or strong attachment to the medial tibial plateau. The medial collateral ligament is often torn along with the medial meniscus.

Lateral meniscus tear.   The lateral meniscus is less frequently injured than the medial meniscus. One possible reason for the lower incidence of injury is the lateral meniscus' greater mobility on the tibial plateau. Greater mobility of the meniscus appears to decrease the stress that is placed on the structure as the joint moves through the range of motion or is subjected to twisting stress.

Patellar Dislocation

Dislocation is usually caused by trauma to the knee, which causes the patella to come out of the central groove on the femur where it usually slides. Symptoms include pain around the patella and difficulty with flexion or extension of the knee joint. Initial treatment of a dislocated patella involves a reduction, or placing the patella back into the correct position.

Another milder form of dislocation is called patellar subluxation. This condition may cause the patella to chronically glide outside its central path. Two factors that may contribute to chronic subluxation are a shallow groove in the femur and patella alta. Patella alta refers to an abnormally high position of the patella in relation to the femur. If the patella is in a position where the groove of the femur is not deep enough, the patella may abnormally track to one side or the other. Most subluxations are in the lateral direction and can be exacerbated by a weak vastus medialis muscle that is unable to hold the patella medially or by a tight iliotibial band or lateral retinaculum that pulls the patella laterally. Physical therapy may be recommended for specific strengthening exercises, and bracing the knee may provide symptomatic relief.

One long-term repercussion to chronic subluxation is the development of chondromalacia patella. As the patella moves in and out of the groove, the cartilage on the underside of the knee is worn down. Therefore, treatment of this condition is similar to the treatment for chondromalacia patella and patellofemoral syndrome. A patella that was previously dislocated is at risk for reinjury. Fitness professionals can design a program for these clients to help reduce the chance of another dislocation. This may include general strengthening of the knee and an emphasis on strengthening the vastus medialis.

Fractures

Fractures can occur with severe knee trauma, such as motor vehicle accidents and contact sports activities. Any of the bones in the knee can be involved. Diagnosis is made through radiographs, and treatment can include prolonged immobilization with casting or other supports or may require surgical repair. After the bone has completely healed, physical therapy may be initiated for strengthening, range of motion exercises, and eventual return to sport. As with all rehabilitation following an injury, the athlete will gradually work into competition after completing sport-specific conditioning exercises and drills.

Study Questions

Complete the following questions. The answer key is on page 107.

1. List four causes of knee pain and injury.

    (1) _____

    (2) _____

    (3) _____

    (4) _____

2. True or false: Chondromalacia patella and patellofemoral syndrome are the same conditions.

3. List two potential causes of patellofemoral syndrome.

    (1) _____

    (2) _____

4. When treating children or adolescents, list four knee conditions the fitness professional should be aware of in this population:

    (1) _____

    (2) _____

    (3) _____

    (4) _____

5. In a survey conducted of high school athletes, which girls and boys sports recorded the highest rates of knee injury.

    boy's _____ and _____

    girl's _____ and _____

6. Fill in the blank: Jumper's knee is also known as _____.

7. List four ways in which the anterior cruciate ligament (ACL) can potentially be injured:

   (1) _____

   (2) _____

   (3) _____

   (4) _____

8. _____, _____, or _____ stress to the knee may also be hazardous to the ACL and cause injury during sporting activities.

9. True or false: Clients who have an ACL tear are predisposed to degenerative changes in the knee joint.

10. True or false: Current scientific evidence supports the recommendation of using an ACL functional knee brace after ACL reconstruction surgery.

11. Name three types of ACL reconstruction surgical techniques:

   (1) _____

   (2) _____

   (3) _____

12. True or false: When matched for activities, females have a greater prevalence for ACL injury than males.

13. It has been hypothesized that some of the differences in injury rate between males and females may be due to limb _____ and _____ differences, sex _____ and _____ laxity, different _____-to-_____ ratios, alterations in muscle _____, movement, and _____ patterns, as well as differences in training.

14. True or false: Scientific studies have shown that a neuromuscular training program can lower the risk of ACL injury in female athletes.

15. List the goals of the PEP program:

    (1) _____

    (2) _____

    (3) _____

    (4) _____

    (5) _____

16. True or false: A posterior cruciate ligament tear can occur when the tibia is forced backward in relation to the femur.

17. The medial collateral ligament is often injured along with which other two structures:

    a. medial and lateral meniscus

    b. medial meniscus and the posterior cruciate ligament

    c. medial meniscus and the anterior cruciate ligament

    d. anterior cruciate ligament and the posterior cruciate ligament

18. List five different types of meniscal tears:

    (1) _____

    (2) _____

    (3) _____

    (4) _____

    (5) _____

19. True or false: The goal of a meniscectomy is to remove as much meniscus as possible in order to form a clean and clear surface inside the joint.

20. True or false: The medial meniscus is torn more frequently than the lateral meniscus because of its decreased mobility, or strong attachment, to the medial tibial plateau.

Chapter 3

Health Screening and Assessment

This chapter outlines your responsibilities as a professional fitness practitioner. It is not meant to be comprehensive but is a reminder that health fitness professionals working with clients who have knee dysfunctions or injuries are responsible for health screening, medical clearance, fitness assessment, exercise monitoring, recordkeeping, emergency procedures, scope of practice, and physician referral.

Health Screening for Physical Activity

Health screening is a crucial first step in maintaining the safety and effectiveness of any exercise program. The purposes of health screening include:

- Identifying health conditions and risk factors that put your client at risk when participating in an exercise program or may necessitate referral to a healthcare professional.
- Assisting in the design of an appropriate exercise program.
- Identifying possible contraindicated activities.
- Fulfilling legal and insurance requirements for you or your facility.
- Encouraging and maintaining communication with the client's healthcare provider.

The Physical Activity Readiness Questionnaire (PAR-Q) has been recommended as a minimal standard for entry into low- to moderate- intensity exercise programs (ACSM 2010; AACVPR 2006). More detailed medical/health history forms may be appropriate for clients with chronic disease or disabilities. A health-screening process is a valuable tool that assists the fitness practitioner in safely and appropriately individualizing the client's exercise program. Information on the form should be referred to often and updated every year or when a change in condition occurs.

Previous Exercise Level and Restrictions

The client assessment should include a history of any surgery, rehabilitation, or other treatment the client has undergone. Some clients who have seen a physical therapist for an injury or rehabilitation after surgery may have continued to use an exercise program designed for them. This will give the fitness professional an idea of what type of training the client has performed and which exercises he or she might already be familiar with. If the client has had surgery, ask when he or she last saw the orthopedic surgeon. It is important to inquire whether the client has been given any specific restrictions from the doctor. If you have any doubts about the appropriate activity level or restrictions for the client, do not hesitate to contact the physician or the physical therapist for guidance.

In addition to the general medical health-screening form, the following knee-specific questions may be helpful in designing a safe and effective exercise program for the knee.

- Have you ever had surgery on the knee, and if so, when?
- What specific type of surgery did you undergo?
- If you had an ACL reconstruction, do you know what type of technique the surgeon used?
- Have you ever been treated by a physical therapist for your knee?
- Has your physician ever given you any specific restrictions? (e.g., running, cutting or pivoting activities)
- When did you last see the orthopedic surgeon who performed your surgery?
- What is your occupation?
- What type of activities or sports do you participate in?
- Do any activities associated with your job or sports aggravate pain in your knee?

Remember that the health-screening process should always be accompanied by careful monitoring and observation during the exercise session.

Re-Entry to Exercise

Clients returning to exercise after injury or surgery may require several weeks to several months to return to their original exercise workloads. They should begin activity at a lesser intensity and gradually progress to higher exercise levels. Re-entry at too rapid a pace can cause reinjury, increased pain, and undesirable stress to the joint.

Medical Clearance

If indicated by the PAR-Q or the health-screening instrument, the client should always be referred to his or her healthcare provider for medical clearance. It is strongly advised that clients with special medical conditions, identified as "at risk," or who are exhibiting symptoms during exercise, obtain medical clearance from his or her physician prior to the start of any exercise program. The American College of Sports Medicine (ACSM) has recommended criteria for situations that warrant a physician's release prior to exercise.

Personal trainers reserve the right to require any participant, upon reviewing his or her medical history, to provide a physician's release prior to undertaking an exercise program. Fitness professionals also might screen individuals who are deemed medically inappropriate from a program. It is important that any physician-signed release that contains specific recommendations, modifications, or restrictions be fully respected and adhered to by the fitness practitioner. Always clarify the maximum limit of exercise and other restrictions with clients and their physicians.

Medications

The health history form should identify any prescription or over-the-counter medications your client is taking. Some medications will influence the heart's response to exercise and your client's exercise tolerance. Others, such as pain relievers, dull pain symptoms that may occur during the exercise program. Be aware of any complaints of pain from the client and modify the exercises appropriately. The Physician's Desk Reference (PDR) is an excellent reference text for more detailed information regarding prescription medications. If you have any questions regarding the client's health history, medical status, medication, or physician's release, contact the physician directly.

Monitoring Exercise

Several effective methods can be used to monitor exercise. Minimum routine monitoring should include heart rate and perceived exertion. In clients with known cardiovascular disease, blood pressure should be monitored.

Heart Rate

The trainer should encourage clients to learn to palpate and count their own heart rate (HR), if possible. However, some clients have lost sensation in the finger pads and may be unable to perform this task. If a client has difficulty finding the pulse at the radial artery, try the temporal artery. The Karvonen formula can be used to establish initial training heart rates.

Perceived Exertion

The BORG Rating of Perceived Exertion (RPE scale) is an acceptable way to monitor exercise intensity and tolerance. This method works well when used in conjunction with HR monitoring. This is the preferred method for clients who are older, returning to exercise from an injury or surgery, on HR-lowering medication, have pain-limiting symptoms, and who are unable to palpate their pulse rate. Perceived exertion is also recommended for clients with exertional angina or claudication and who are extremely deconditioned. The RPE should be compatible with the client's physical appearance and response to the exercise.

Pain Scale

A pain scale from 0 to 10 can be used to rate the client's discomfort with exercise, with 0 indicating no pain and 10 indicating pain so severe the client would need to go to the emergency room. Pain level varies greatly among people. A mild to moderate pain level is not acceptable during fitness training. If a client experiences pain of this severity, he or she should be referred to a physician.

Physical Symptoms of Overwork

Practitioners, as well as clients, should be taught to observe physical signs and symptoms that indicate overwork. Signs of overwork include:

- Abnormal musculoskeletal pain or discomfort
- Elevated heart rate that is above what is normal for the client
- Red face
- Abnormal shortness of breath with exercise
- Excessive perspiration
- Abnormal fatigue
- Chest pain or palpitations
- Excessive fatigue or discomfort

In addition, clients should be instructed not to exercise during an acute illness, when fatigued, or under excessive stress. Clients should be taught to identify and report any inappropriate responses to exercise.

Recordkeeping

Recordkeeping is an integral part of any exercise program and is important to demonstrate objective improvement to the client, practitioner, and healthcare provider. It assists in guiding the progression of exercise and is helpful in determining normal and abnormal responses to exercise. This is particularly true for heart rate and blood pressure responses at rest and during exercise, as well as musculoskeletal pain or fatigue that may occur during or after exercise. If the client were to have any problem during or after exercise, documentation of exercise progression and tolerance would be important. Any changes in medication or physician recommendations should be noted and adhered to.

Be sure to record in the client's daily workout log any abnormal responses to exercise. A client whose function is not maintained or who does not improve with adequate adherence to appropriate exercise may require physician evaluation.

Scope of Practice

It is vitally important for your client's safety and your own to work within the limits and scope of your professional training and qualifications. Performing therapeutic treatments, recommending dietary changes or nutritional supplements for the treatment of joint disease, or modifying a client's prescribed medication dosage are just a few of the tasks that are beyond an exercise practitioner's scope of practice. Only a physician can diagnose and treat a knee injury. Refer your client to a medical professional if you are ever uncertain of an underlying injury or knee condition. Upon release from the physician to exercise or upon completion of physical therapy, the fitness professional can be an integral part of a person's return to physical activity and training following an injury to the knee.

Risk Management

Every fitness professional must have a risk-management plan to ensure the safety and effectiveness of the exercise program. A basic risk-management plan includes the following: (1) identification of risk areas; (2) evaluation of specific risks in each area; (3) selection of appropriate treatment for each risk; (4) implementation of a risk-management system; and (5) evaluation of success. In addition, risk management includes establishing contact with your client's healthcare team, knowing when to refer your client to his or her physician, and knowing and following emergency procedures.

Emergency Procedures

It is important to know emergency medical procedures and have a system in place for responding to a medical emergency. An emergency plan must be in place for every training situation. In a medical emergency, act quickly and insist on prompt medical attention, even if the client resists.

If your client has a history of cardiac disease, pay close attention to their symptoms. Pain in the left shoulder could be an indication of a heart attack in progress. When in doubt, call 911. While waiting for emergency medical services to arrive, keep the person quiet, in a half-sitting position, and try to relieve his or her anxiety. Loosen clothing and maintain an even body temperature. Do not lift the person or give him food or drink. If the person is unconscious:

- Check breathing. If the person is not breathing, and if you are qualified to do so, initiate artificial respiration.
- Check for a heartbeat. If the person is not breathing and there is no pulse, initiate CPR until medical help arrives, but only if you are trained to perform CPR.
- If your worksite has an automated external defibrillator (AED) and you have been trained in its use, use it.

Emergency treatment aims to restore normal heartbeat and blood flow as quickly as possible. Once the person is in the hands of a trained medical professional, medications will be administered to stabilize heart rate and blood pressure and to relieve pain. The person may be treated with:

- Pain relievers
- Medications that control blood pressure and heart rhythms
- Medications to relax the patient and reduce the stress of the event
- Oxygen
- Defibrillation or electric shock, which may be necessary to restore or correct the heartbeat

Throughout the medical treatment process there is continuous monitoring of all vital signs.

Physician Contact and Referral

Establishing contact and developing rapport with the medical community will greatly enhance your ability to provide for your clients. Maintaining relationships with healthcare providers ensures a safe program for clients and establishes credibility with physicians and healthcare professionals. A relationship between you and the medical community also builds a referral system and is an excellent way for the physician and fitness professional to exchange education information.

Inappropriate responses to exercise that are persistent, that indicate termination of exercise, or that occur consistently require the client to be referred to his or her physician or healthcare provider. If there is ever any doubt about the appropriateness of exercise, check with your medical advisor or the client's physician.

Client Assessment

The following tests can be performed on any client to determine knee range of motion, flexibility, strength, stability, and balance. Results from the assessment can be used to plan an appropriate fitness program as well as measure progress in these areas. The tests provide a general assessment and are not meant to be used for clinical diagnosis. If range of motion or strength is severely affected, or if pain is caused by any of these tests, referral of the client to a medical professional is warranted.

Range of Motion

Adequate knee range of motion is necessary for proper ambulation and other activities, such as squatting. Flexibility of the muscles surrounding the knee joint is also required. Range of motion can be affected by loose structures within the joint itself, such as torn cartilage or bony fragments. It can also be reduced from swelling that is present inside or around the knee. For instance, a flap from a torn meniscus can block the full extension of the knee joint, or swelling and edema may cause the client to be unable to bend the knee into flexion.

Normal knee joint extension measures approximately 0 degrees, meaning the knee is fully straightened. Knee flexion for the normal client should be around 130 degrees. Figures 3.1 and 3.2 (page 44) illustrate normal and decreased knee range of motion.

Evaluating the range of motion may also indicate which muscles require flexibility training. If the knee were 30 degrees away from being straight, it would be important to stretch the hamstring muscles as part of the client's program. Likewise, if there is no history of injury and the knee only bends to 90 degrees, the flexibility of the quadriceps should be addressed. Figures 3.3 and 3.4 (pages 45–46) show a client with normal and decreased flexibility.

Recording the approximate joint range of motion during the assessment will help track the client's progress throughout the training sessions. In addition, always check the range of motion on both sides to see if they are equal and how far away the client is from the norm.

Figure 3.1. Knee extension

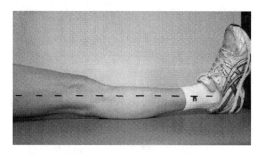

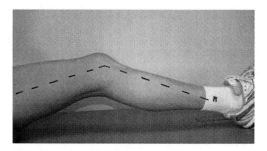

Normal range of motion   Decreased range of motion

Figure 3.2. Knee Flexion

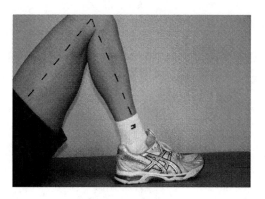

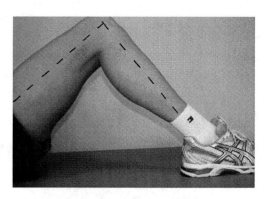

Normal range of motion   Decreased range of motion

Muscle Flexibility

Information about muscle flexibility is important to gain during an assessment because muscle imbalances may lead to gait deviations and affect the function of the knee. The two most important muscle groups to test are the quadriceps and the hamstrings.

Quadriceps Flexibility Test

Positioning   Lie prone on a table.

Movement   Keeping the hips level, slowly bend the knee toward the buttocks until resistance is felt. The client should avoid trunk rotation, arching of the back, or allowing the test leg to come up off the table.

Interpretation   Normally the client should be close to touching the heel to the buttocks. An objective measurement can be taken by recording the number of inches between the heel and the buttocks. Compare both sides for discrepancies and take note if the client experiences any discomfort. Figure 3.3 shows normal flexibility and inflexibility of the quadriceps muscles. Always test both sides for comparison. This measurement can be taken again after an exercise program of stretching the quadriceps is initiated.

Figure 3.3. Quadriceps flexibility test

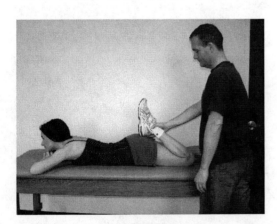

Normal flexibility

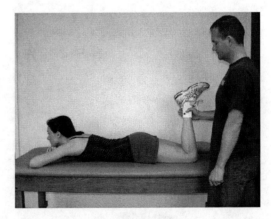

Inflexibility

Hamstrings Flexibility Test

Positioning   Lie supine on a table.

Movement   Keeping the test knee straight and the low back flat on the table, lift up the leg until resistance is felt. The client should avoid bending the knee or allowing the back to arch off the table. Keep the foot relaxed to avoid involvement of the gastrocnemius muscle. In addition, the opposite leg should be maintained in extension and remain flat on the table during the testing. It may be necessary to stabilize this leg by applying gentle pressure to the front of the thigh, just above the knee. If the knee starts to bend, lower the leg slightly so the knee is able to fully extend. Estimate the degree of angle between the elevated leg and the table. A position of 90 degrees is representative of the leg being directly perpendicular to the table.

Interpretation   Normal hamstring length is considered to be around 80 degrees. Compare both sides for discrepancies and take note if the client experiences any discomfort. Figure 3.4 shows normal flexibility and inflexibility of the hamstring muscles. Always test both sides for comparison. This measurement can be taken again after an exercise program of stretching the hamstrings is initiated.

Figure 3.4. Hamstrings flexibility test

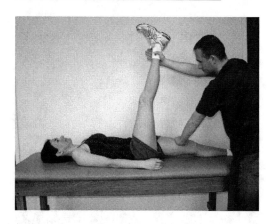

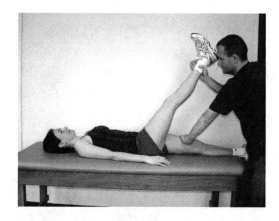

Normal flexibility   Inflexibility

Strength

Strength is one of the most important fitness components to assess. The knee is one of the main weight-bearing joints in the body. Without proper strength a person cannot walk properly, transfer in and out of a chair easily, or balance accurately. The following tests give the fitness professional an idea of the client's strength in the knee.

Quadriceps Strength Test

Positioning   Sitting on the edge of a table or in a chair.
Movement   Place one hand over the ankle and stabilize the thigh with your other hand. Have the client attempt to straighten the leg against the resistance.
Interpretation   A client who lacks full quadriceps strength may not be able to push strongly enough to move the resisting hand away. Compare both sides and take note if the client experiences any discomfort.

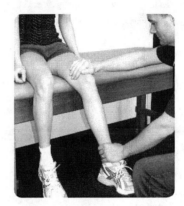

Hamstrings Strength Test

Positioning   Sitting on the edge of a table or in a chair.
Movement   Place one hand behind the client's lower leg and stabilize the thigh with your other hand. The client begins the test with the leg slightly extended and then attempts to bend the knee against the resistance.
Interpretation   A client who lacks full hamstring strength may not be able to pull strongly enough to move the resisting hand toward the table. Compare both sides and take note if the client experiences any discomfort.

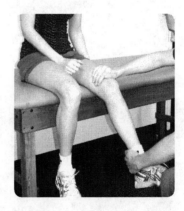

If knee pain is experienced during any of these tests, it may indicate inflammation or other musculoskeletal conditions and should be evaluated by a physician or physical therapist before initiating an exercise program.

One Repetition Maximum

The one repetition maximum (1-RM) is a test that determines the maximum amount of weight the client can move for one repetition while maintaining proper form. The 1-RM should be performed **only** on healthy clients who are not experiencing pain and have not undergone knee surgery. There are a number of 1-RM calculators that estimate the 1-RM value by plugging the number of repetitions (< 10) and the weight lifted into a formula. The 1-RM is an objective way to gauge an individual's muscle strength. One formula used to calculate the 1-RM is:

$$\frac{\text{Amount of Weight Lifted}}{1.0278 - (.0278 \times \text{Number of Reps})} = 1\text{-RM}$$

To calculate, multiply 0.0278 by the number of repetitions completed to the point of fatigue. Subtract the answer (the product) from 1.0278. Take the weight lifted and divide it by the previous answer. The result is the 1-RM, or the estimated maximum weight the client can lift once with proper form. This test can be used to test lower extremity strength with the squat or deadlift. The 1-RM is just an estimate, but it provides the fitness professional with one way of objectively documenting gains in a client's exercise program.

There are other ways in which you can measure a client's progress with strength other than performing a specific test. One way is to ask the client how he or she is using the leg functionally. Is the client able to walk or run for longer distances? Does he or she have any difficulty with stair climbing? Is he or she playing recreational sports with greater ability? Does the leg feel more stable when standing on it? The client is a good source of information regarding subjective progress.

Another indication of strength gains is the amount of weight the client is able to use during the exercise routine. It does not have to be a great deal of weight to indicate an increase in strength. A client may have started his or her routine using 1 lb ankle weights for 2 sets of 10 repetitions and is now able to perform the same exercises with 3 lb ankle weights for 3 sets of 10 repetitions. Similarly, the client may now be using a resistive band of greater strength. A stronger blue band may have taken the place of an easier yellow band for knee strengthening exercises.

Girth Measurement

A circumferential measurement taken around the thigh is an easy way of estimating the girth of the underlying musculature. Muscle atrophy can be subtle, so taking an objective measurement may help to quantify this loss of muscle girth.

Position   Standing with weight evenly distributed between both feet and the legs slightly apart.

Measurement   To measure the muscle girth, wrap a tape measure around the thigh approximately 5 inches above the knee joint line. Make sure the tape measure is not too tight or too loose and is held in a horizontal position across the thigh.

Interpretation   Measure both thighs for comparison. Be aware that swelling around the knee and adipose tissue can interfere with a true reading of the muscle girth. This measurement can be taken again after a strengthening program is initiated.

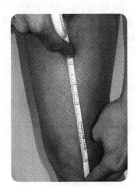 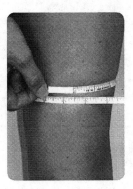

Single-Leg Stability

The fitness professional can evaluate both the client's stability and balance by having him or her perform this simple test on each leg.

Position   Standing upright on one leg with both arms at the sides. Bend the non-weight-bearing leg to 90 degrees.

Measurement   The client slowly descends into a squatting position with the weight-bearing knee at 30–40 degrees of flexion. Repeat up to 10 times while keeping good posture and staying upright. The knee should not go beyond the toes when testing. Figure 3.5 shows the correct testing positions.

Interpretation   The client should be able to perform this mini squat 10 times without placing the opposite foot on the ground for balance and without abnormal movements such as caving in of the leg or allowing the trunk to come into flexion. Figure 3.6 shows abnormal movements made during the Single-Leg Stability test. Test both sides for comparison. This test can be performed again after a strengthening program is initiated.

Figure 3.5. Single-leg stability test

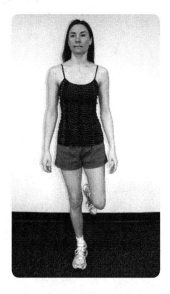 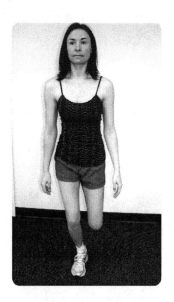 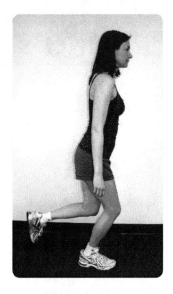

Starting test position   Ending test position   Side view

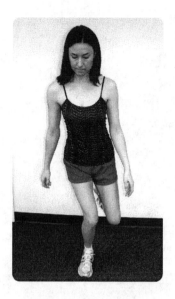

Caving in of the leg

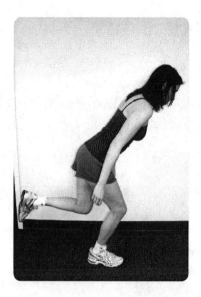

Trunk flexion

Figure 3.6. Abnormal test movements

Gait Pattern

After undergoing a knee surgery, a client may have some form of ambulation abnormality. An ambulation abnormality can be due to muscle weakness, a loss of range of motion, continued pain in the limb, or a developed habit. Some clients will not have any visible deficits, but muscular testing will indicate weakness in the knee. A note should be made about any type of gait pattern abnormality when first meeting with a client.

An antalgic gait pattern is one in which the person limps, usually due to pain. The person does not put full weight on the limb and quickly transfers the weight off the involved leg. The fitness professional should be able to pick out this abnormality when watching clients walk. If the client experiences pain with walking, a referral should be made for this client to see a physician or physical therapist.

Study Questions

Complete the following questions. The answer key is on page 108.

1. List three questions specific to the client's knee that may be helpful in designing a safe and effective exercise program.

   (1) _____

   (2) _____

   (3) _____

2. List three purposes for health screening.

   (1) _____

   (2) _____

   (3) _____

3. List three appropriate ways to monitor exercise.

   (1) _____

   (2) _____

   (3) _____

4. True or false: Normal knee flexion is 90 degrees and normal knee extension is 0 degrees.

5. True or false: The strength of the quadriceps muscle is tested by asking the client to bend the knee against the resistance of the fitness professional's hand.

6. True or false: If knee pain is experienced during any of type of testing, it may indicate inflammation or other musculoskeletal conditions, and should be evaluated by a physician or physical therapist before initiating an exercise program.

7. The _____ test allows the fitness professional to evaluate both the client's stability and balance.

Chapter 4

Exercises

This chapter explains in detail the exercises that are appropriate for increasing the strength and flexibility of the knee joint. Each exercise is broken down into a description of the starting position, the movements and muscles involved, common errors made while performing the exercise, and reminders to give the client for maintaining proper form. Finally, modifications are provided to progress the client as needed. All exercises should be performed in a slow and controlled manner.

Training Principles

When planning an exercise routine for clients, it is important to remember a few principles regarding resistive weight, repetitions, speed, and type of contraction. It is also imperative to adjust your program for clients who may be returning to exercise following injury or surgery to the knee.

Some additional principles of training include:

- Warm up for at least 5 minutes before starting the strengthening or flexibility routine.
- Build slowly: Do not overload muscles too quickly. At the end of 10–15 repetitions the muscles should feel slightly fatigued. If the exercise is too easy, increase the number of repetitions or add more weight.
- Move slowly and smoothly: Do not jerk or use momentum to complete the exercises. Take a few seconds to perform each stage of the exercise. For

example, lift for a count of 3 seconds, hold for 2 seconds, and then lower
to a count of 3.
- Breathe: Don't hold the breath while exercising. Exhale during the exertion, and inhale while returning to the starting point.
- Use proper posture: When performing squats, knee bends, and lunges,
never allow the knees to pass over the toes. Performing these exercises with
the knees past the toes increases the stress on the knee joint and potentially
causes injury.

Weight and Repetitions

Begin new exercises without weight or with very light resistance. In general, as the weight
increases, the repetitions decrease. Gradually increase to 2 to 3 sets of 10 repetitions.
When the exercise becomes easier, increase the weight and decrease the repetitions.

Speed

To get the most from the exercises it is best to perform the repetitions slowly. Caution
must be used to ensure the exercise is performed correctly and with proper form.

Concentric versus Eccentric

Concentric movement is one in which the muscle is contracting into a shortened position. A concentric exercise is usually performed against gravity. An example is straightening your knee while sitting in a chair. The quadriceps muscles are contracting and
their length is shortened. Another example is the knee-straightening portion of the squat
exercise. When the clients straighten their knees and come to an upright position, the
quadriceps are working concentrically.

   An eccentric contraction is one in which the muscle is contracting, but at the same
time being lengthened. This contraction usually slows the movement against gravity.
Turning again to the squat exercise, as the knees are bent and the body is lowered toward the ground, the quadriceps are contracting eccentrically to allow a slow, controlled
descent of the body. If the quadriceps were not contracting, the body would fall toward
the ground. Eccentric contractions require greater muscle effort than concentric contractions. Performing eccentric contractions in a slow, controlled manner increases the training challenge.

Open Kinetic Chain versus Closed Kinetic Chain

The human body functions as an interconnected series of segments, or a kinetic chain,
that is linked through joints, muscles, and other stabilizing structures. Exercises can be
classified as either open or closed kinetic chain activities. Understanding the differences

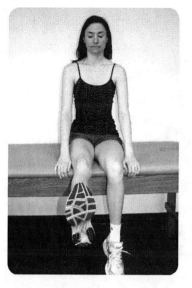
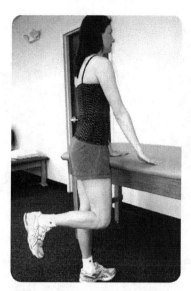

Leg Kick-Out   Hamstring Curl

Figure 4.1. Open kinetic chain exercises

between the two types of exercises can help the fitness professional choose the safest and most appropriate activities for their client's training routine.

Open kinetic chain exercises are those in which the foot is not in contact with a solid surface. In other words, the distal segment, or the foot, is free to move without resistance. Open kinetic chain exercises usually isolate a single muscle group or a single joint and can be performed with or without added weight. Figure 4.1 shows examples of open kinetic chain exercises.

Closed kinetic chain exercises are those in which the foot is in a constant fixed position, usually on the ground or in a weight-bearing position. These types of exercises involve multiple muscle groups and joints. Closed kinetic chain exercises can be performed with the body weight alone or with added weight. Figure 4.2 shows examples of closed kinetic chain exercises.

Research has shown that open kinetic chain exercises produce significantly greater shear forces at the knee joint than closed kinetic chain exercises (Lutz et al. 1993). This finding has potential implications when designing an exercise routine for clients with knee injuries, such as an ACL tear, or degenerative conditions, such as osteoarthritis.

Closed kinetic chain exercises are thought to be more functional because they often mimic activities that we perform on a daily basis or during sports activities. In 1993, Lutz et al. demonstrated that closed kinetic chain exercises produce greater compressive

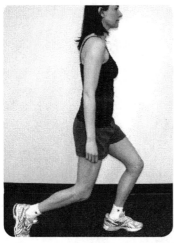

Lunge

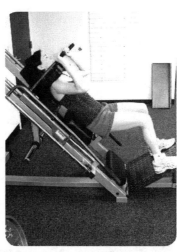

Leg press machine

Figure 4.2. Closed kinetic chain exercises

forces than open kinetic chain exercises and create increased muscular co-contraction at the knee joint. This increase in compression helps stabilize the knee and assists in strengthening the muscles surrounding the joint, such as the hamstrings and quadriceps. Furthermore, a study in 2003 by Stensdotter et al. demonstrated that "exercise in closed kinetic chain promotes more balanced initial quadriceps activation than does exercise in open kinetic chain" (pg. 2043). In this study the vastus medialis muscle was recruited last in the open kinetic chain exercise, which may be of importance when designing a training program for individuals with patellofemoral problems.

Strengthening Exercises

The exercises in this section are organized into beginner, intermediate, and advanced. The primary muscles that are used in each exercise are listed, the positioning and execution of the exercises are described, and any client reminders or common mistakes are provided. Finally, modifications are provided to progress the client as needed.

Beginner Exercises

The exercises in this section are the easiest to perform; however, most can be progressed to a more challenging level. These exercises can also be used for clients who are deconditioned or who have not exercised in awhile.

Resistance Band Quadriceps Push   quadriceps

Positioning   Sit on a mat with one leg partially bent. Place a resistive band under the knee and hold on to both ends of the band with one hand.

Execution   Push the knee down and straighten the leg. Hold for 5 seconds.

Client reminders   Hold the band tight and do not allow your hand to move. Repeat on the other side.

Modification   Increase the resistance of the band or place more tension on the band prior to initiating the movement.

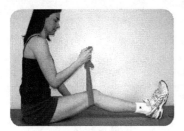   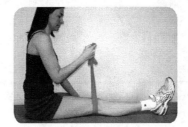

Starting position   Ending position

Pillow Squeeze   quadriceps, especially the vastus medialis

Positioning   Lie on your back or supported by your arms, with both knees straight. Place a folded pillow or small ball between the knees.

Execution   Push the knee down to straighten the leg and then squeeze the pillow with both legs. Hold for 5 seconds.

Client reminders   Keep both knees straight.

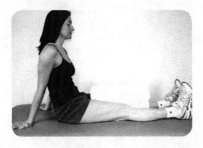

Straight-Leg Lift   quadriceps

Positioning   Lie on your back or propped on the elbows, with one leg straight and the opposite knee bent.
Execution   Keeping the knee straight, lift the leg approximately 12 inches off the mat. Hold for 5 seconds.
Client reminder   Keep the leg straight. Repeat on the other side.
Common error   Allowing the knee to bend and lifting primarily with the hip flexors.
Modifications   Add ankle weights to make the exercise more challenging.

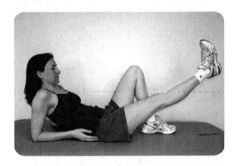

Straight-Leg Lift with Toe Out   quadriceps, especially the vastus medialis

Positioning   Lie on your back or propped on elbows. Straighten one knee and turn the toe outward. Keep the opposite knee bent.
Execution   Keeping the knee straight, lift the leg approximately 12 inches off the mat. Hold for 5 seconds.
Client reminder   Keep the leg straight. Repeat on the other side.
Common error   Allowing the knee to bend and lifting primarily with the hip flexors.
Modifications   Add ankle weights to make the exercise more challenging.

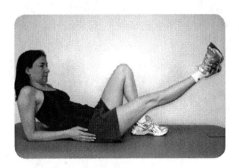

Leg Kick-Out   quadriceps

Positioning Sit on a table or in a chair.
Execution Straighten the knee fully and hold for 5 seconds. Slowly lower the leg back to the starting position.
Client reminder Keep the thigh supported. Repeat on the other side.
Modification Add ankle weights to make the exercise more challenging. Use leg extension machine.

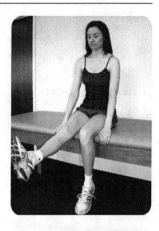

Sidelying Abduction   quadriceps, especially the vastus lateralis

Positioning Lie on your side. Bend the bottom knee and keep the upper knee straight.
Execution Lift the straight leg off the bottom leg. Hold for 5 seconds.
Client reminders Keep the leg straight. Do not let the hips drop forward or backward. Repeat on the other side.
Modification Add ankle weights to make the exercise more challenging.

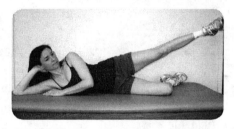

Sidelying Adduction   quadriceps, especially the vastus medialis

Positioning Lie on your side. Place the sole of the top foot behind the straightened bottom leg.
Execution Lift the bottom leg up off the mat. Hold for 5 seconds.
Client reminders Keep the leg straight. Do not let the hips drop forward or backward. Repeat on the other side.
Modification Use a stool or foam roller and

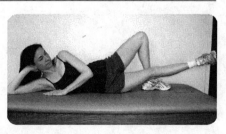

place the upper leg on top of it. Add ankle weights to make the exercise more challenging.

Standing Hamstring Curl   hamstrings

Positioning   Stand with feet shoulder-width apart. Use a support for balance if needed.
Execution   Bend one knee to approximately 90 degrees. Slowly lower the foot back to the floor.
Client reminders   Keep back straight and contract the abdominals. Repeat on the other side.
Modifications   Add ankle weights to make the exercise more challenging. Use leg curl machine.

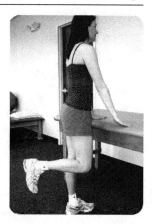

Bridges on Ball   hamstrings

Positioning   Lie on your back and place both calves on top of a stability ball.
Execution   Lift hips off floor. Slowly lower to starting position.
Client reminders   Keep hips level and do not allow one side to drop. Do not push down with the arms.
Modifications   Place the ball under the ankles or use one leg only.

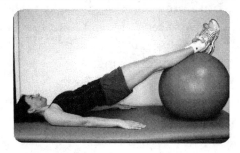

Intermediate Exercises

These exercises are for clients who require more of a challenge or who have mastered the beginner exercises. When performing any type of squatting or lunging exercise, it is extremely important to keep the knees from passing over the toes. Figure 4.3 shows the proper positioning of the knees during the squat and lunge exercise. Figure 4.4 shows improper positioning of the knees.

Figure 4.3. Proper positioning of the knees

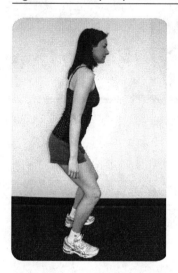 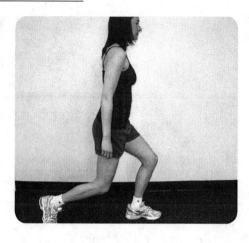

Figure 4.4. Improper positioning of the knees: knees past toes

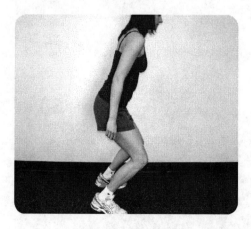 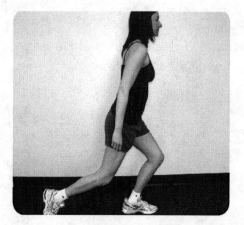

Standing Knee Extension with Resistance Band   quadriceps

Positioning   Stand with the resistance band around the upper portion of the calf with the other portion of the band attached to something sturdy. Begin with the knee slightly bent.

Execution   Straighten the knee against the resistance of the band.

Client reminders   Do not lean your body back when straightening the leg. Repeat on the other side.

Common error   Pulling back with the hip and not the knee.

Modification   Increase the resistance of the band or place more tension on the band prior to initiating the movement.

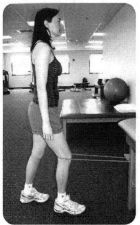 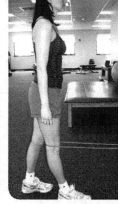

Starting position   Ending position

Hamstring Curls with Resistance Band   hamstrings

Positioning   Sit on a chair or stool with the resistance band around the lower calf or ankle and the other portion of the band attached to something sturdy. Begin with the knee slightly bent.

Execution   Bend the knee against the resistance of the band to approximately 90 degrees.

Client reminders   Keep the hips level and do not raise the buttocks. Repeat on the other side.

Modification   Increase the resistance of the band or place more tension on the band prior to initiating the movement.

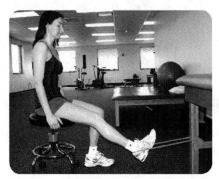 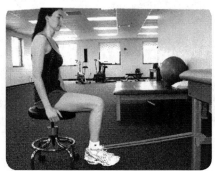

Starting position   Ending position

Resistance Band Leg Pulls

Positioning   Stand with the resistance band around the ankle and the other portion of the band attached to something sturdy. Use a support for balance if needed.

Execution   This exercise can be performed in four different directions: hip flexion, hip extension, hip abduction, and hip adduction.

Client reminders   Stand straight and do not lean forward or to the side. Keep the knee of the active leg straight but not locked. Keep the toes of the active leg pointing upward. Repeat on the other side.

Common errors   Bending the knee of the active leg. Leaning forward while pulling the band back.

Modification   Increase the resistance of the band or place more tension on the band prior to initiating the movement. Use the multi-hip weight machine or weight stack with ankle cuff attachment.

Note   The client will often feel a greater strain on the leg they are standing on than the leg they are pulling the band with.

Flexion   quadriceps

Execution   Pull band forward, keeping the knee straight.

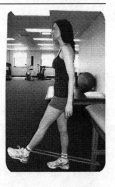

Extension   quadriceps, hamstrings

Execution   Pull band backward, keeping the knee straight.

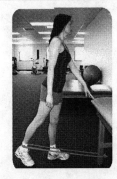

Abduction   quadriceps, especially the vastus lateralis

Execution   Pull band out to the side, keeping the knee straight.

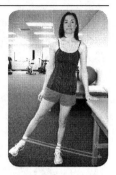

Adduction   quadriceps, especially the vastus medialis

Execution   Pull band in toward midline, keeping knee straight.

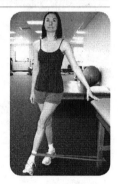

Wall Squats   quadriceps

Positioning   Rest the back on the wall with both feet approximately 2–3 feet from the wall.

Execution   Slide the back down the wall and hold for 5 seconds. Straighten both knees and slide back to starting position.

Client reminder   Do not let the knees pass over the toes. Do not go past a 90-degree angle.

Modifications

- Use a stability ball behind the small of the back when sliding down the wall to reduce friction.
- Hold the squat for a longer amount of time (e.g., 20–30 seconds each).
- Hold dumbbells in each hand.
- Instruct the client to perform a set of 6 squats. The first is held for 10 seconds, the second squat for 20 seconds, and so forth. The sixth or last squat is held for a full 60 seconds.
- To emphasize the vastus medialis, turn the toes out to a 45-degree angle.
- Step away from the wall and perform the squat without back support.

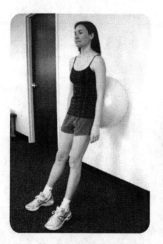

Starting position

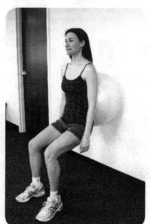

Ending position

Resistance Band Squats   quadriceps

Positioning   Stand on a resistance band with feet shoulder-width apart. Hold onto the ends of the band.

Execution   Bend knees while holding the band in the same position. Straighten knees slowly against the resistance of the band. Keep back flat and contract the abdominals.

Common error   Losing tension in the band during the exercise.

Modifications   Increase the resistance of the band or place more tension on the band prior to initiating the movement. To emphasize the vastus medialis, turn the toes out to a 45-degree angle.

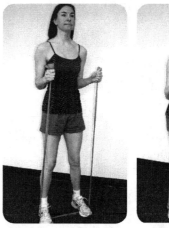
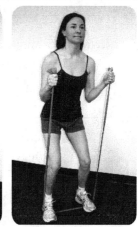

Starting position   Ending position

Step-Ups   quadriceps

Positioning   Stand with the box in front of you for forward direction; on top of the box for backward; or to the side of the box for lateral step-ups.

Execution   This exercise can be performed in three different directions: forward, backward, and lateral.

Modification   Increase the height of the step or box.

Client reminder   Repeat on the other side.

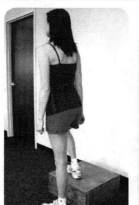
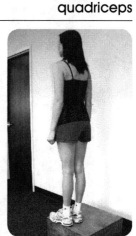

Lateral starting position   Laeral ending position

Stool Pulls   hamstrings

Positioning   Sit on a rolling stool with knees bent at a 90-degree angle and feet flat on the floor.

Execution   Straighten one knee and then dig the heel into the floor, pulling the stool forward. Alternate legs.

Modification   Use both legs at the same time, or use one leg only. Increase the distance. For more resistance, roll stool on carpet rather than linoleum or tile.

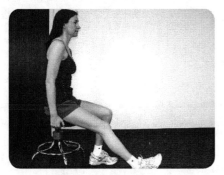
Starting position

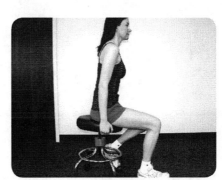
Ending position

Sideways Squat Walk with Resistance Band   quadriceps

Positioning   Place a resistance band, tied in a knot, around the lower legs. Squat slightly and do not allow the knees to pass over the toes.

Execution   Step sideways with the band kept tight and the knees bent.

Client reminder   Stay in a squatting position, take large steps, and keep the band tight. Do not allow the knees to pass over the toes.

Modification   Increase the resistance of the band or place more tension on the band prior to initiating the movement. Increase the distance.

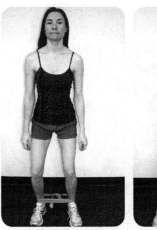
Starting position

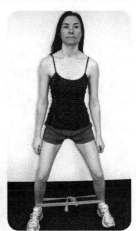
Ending position

Forward Lunge   quadriceps and hamstrings

Positioning   Stand with feet together.
Execution   Step forward with one foot and bend the
knee. Allow the trailing knee to drop toward the floor.
Client reminder   Do not allow the front knee to pass
over the toes. Repeat on the other side.
Modifications
  • Hold dumbbells in each hand while performing
    the exercise.
  • Place the front foot on half-round or full-round
    foam roller.
  • Alternate legs and walk forward.

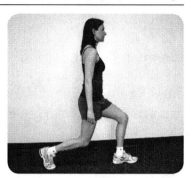

Lunge with Back Leg on Ball   quadriceps and hamstrings

Positioning   Stand with one foot in front of the other. Place the back foot on a stability
ball.
Execution   Bend the front knee and allow the trailing knee to drop toward the floor.
Client reminders   Do not allow the front knee to pass over the toes. Keep weight balanced over the front foot. Repeat on the other side.
Modification   Hold dumbbells in each hand while performing the exercise.

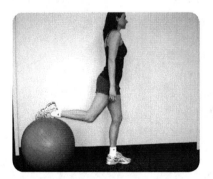
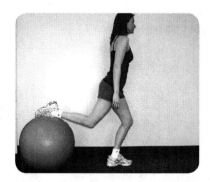

Starting position   Ending position

Backward Lunge
quadriceps, with emphasis on the trailing leg

Positioning   Stand with feet together.

Execution   Step backward with one foot in a lunge position and allow both knees to bend.

Client reminders   Do not allow the front knee to pass over the toes. Keep weight centered over the trailing leg. Repeat on the other side.

Modification   Hold dumbbells in each hand while performing the exercise.

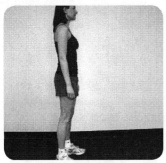
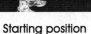
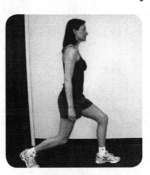

Starting position   Ending position

Hamstring Curl and Kick
hamstrings

Positioning   Lean over the edge of a table.

Execution   First, bend one knee to a 90-degree angle, then lift from the hip while extending the leg behind the body.

Client reminders   Do not arch the back when lifting the leg. Repeat on the other side.

Common error   Performing both movements at once. Twisting the trunk while extending the hip.

Modification   Add ankle weights to make the exercise more challenging.

Note   Do not perform this exercise if the client experiences back pain.

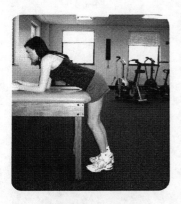
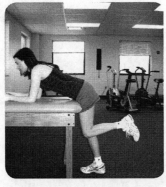
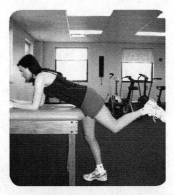

Starting position   Second position   Ending position

Advanced Exercises

These exercises are for clients who have been training regularly and are able to withstand a greater challenge. Do not have the client perform these exercises if he or she experiences pain.

Step Dips   quadriceps

Positioning   Stand on a step or box. Use support for balance if needed.

Execution   While standing on one leg, squat slightly until the heel or toe of the opposite foot is touching the floor. Immediately straighten the leg on the step so weight is not placed on the foot touching the floor.

Client reminders   Do not transfer the weight to the foot touching the floor. Repeat on the other side.

Modification   Increase the height of the step to make the exercise more challenging.

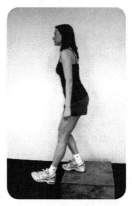
Forward ending
position

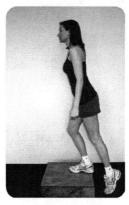
Backward ending
position

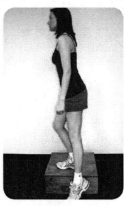
Lateral ending
position

Lunge and Lift   quadriceps and hamstrings

Positioning   Begin with both feet together. Lunge forward with one foot in front of the other and both knees bent.

Execution   Straighten the front leg while at the same time lifting the back leg off the floor. Lower the back leg and return to the starting position.

Client reminder   Stand up straight and contract your abdominals. Do not use your back leg to push off. Repeat on the other side.

Modifications

- Hold dumbbells in each hand while performing the exercise.
- Alternate legs and walk forward.
- Place a weight around the ankle.

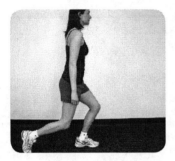
Starting position

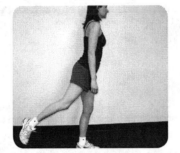
Ending position

Leg Kick-Out on Ball   quadriceps and hamstrings

Positioning   Lie with back supported by stability ball. Keep the hips elevated, knees bent at a 90-degree angle, and feet flat on the floor.

Execution   Lift one foot and straighten the leg until it is parallel to the floor.

Client reminders   Keep the thighs parallel to the floor. Do not allow the hips to sag. Keep the low back stabilized on the ball. Repeat on the other side.

Modification   Place a weight around the ankle.

Note   Do not perform this exercise if the client experiences back pain.

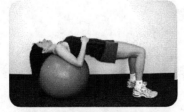
Starting position

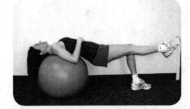
Ending position

Hamstring Curls on Ball   hamstrings

Positioning   Lie on your back with knees straight and heels on a stability ball. Lift hips off the floor.

Execution   Bend knees and bring ball toward buttocks. Straighten knees out to starting position.

Modifications   Perform the exercise with only one leg while keeping the opposite knee straight.

Note   Do not perform this exercise if the client experiences back pain.

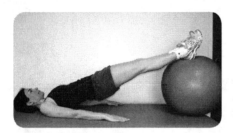

Starting position

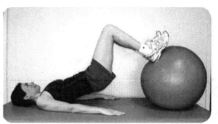

Ending position

Single-Leg Wall Squats   quadriceps

Positioning   Rest the back on the wall with both feet approximately 2–3 feet from the wall. Lift one foot off the floor.

Execution   Slide the back down the wall and hold for 5 seconds. Straighten the knee and slide back to starting position.

Client reminder   Do not let the knee pass over the toes. Repeat on the other side.

Modifications

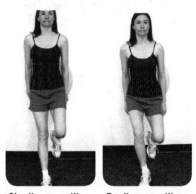

Starting position   Ending position

- Use a stability ball behind the small of the back when sliding down the wall to reduce friction.
- Hold the squat for a longer amount of time (e.g., 20–30 seconds each).
- Hold dumbbells in each hand.
- Instruct the client to perform a set of 6 squats. The first is held for 10 seconds, the second squat for 20 seconds, and so forth. The sixth or last squat is held for a full 60 seconds.
- To emphasize the vastus medialis, turn the toe on the standing leg out to a 45-degree angle.
- Step away from the wall and perform squat without back support.

Resistance Band Single-Leg Squats — quadriceps

Positioning   Stand on a resistance band with feet shoulder-width apart. Hold on to the ends of the band. Lift one foot off the floor.

Execution   Bend knee while holding the band in the same position. Straighten knee slowly against the resistance of the band.

Client reminders   Do not allow the knee to pass over the toes. Keep your back straight and contract the abdominals. Repeat on the other side.

Common error   Losing tension in the band during the exercise.

Modification   Increase the resistance of the band or place more tension on the band prior to initiating the movement. To emphasize the vastus medialis, turn the toe out to a 45-degree angle.

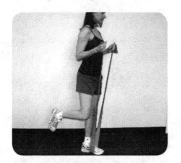 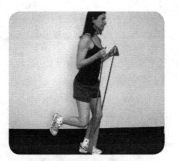

Starting position   Ending position

Resistance Band Lunge — quadriceps and hamstrings

Positioning   Stand with one foot in front of the other and a resistance band under the front foot. Hold on to the ends of the band.

Execution   Bend the front knee and allow the trailing knee to drop toward the floor. Keep the band held in the same position. Straighten the knee slowly against the resistance of the band.

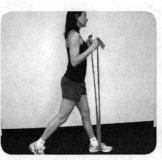 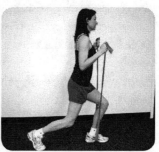

Starting position   Ending position

Client reminder   Do not allow the front knee to pass over the toes. Keep your back straight and contract the abdominals. Repeat on the other side.

Common error   Losing tension in the band during the exercise.

Modification   Increase the resistance of the band or place more tension on the band prior to initiating the movement.

Foam Roller Squats   quadriceps

Positioning   Stand on a half-round foam roller with the flat side down and the feet shoulder-width apart.
Execution   Bend the knees slightly, then return to the starting position.
Client reminders   Do not allow the knees to pass over the toes. Keep the back straight and contract the abdominals.
Modifications
  • Increase the challenge by turning the foam roller over and standing on the flat side.
  • Perform single-leg squats on the half-round foam roller.
  • Progress to standing on a full-round foam roller.
  • Hold dumbbells in each hand.

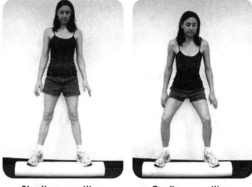

Starting position   Ending position

Foam Roller Lunges   quadriceps and hamstrings

Positioning   Stand on a half-round foam roller with the flat side down and one foot in front of the other.
Execution   Bend the front knee and allow the trailing knee to drop toward the floor.
Client reminder   Do not allow the front knee to pass over the toes.
Modifications   Hold dumbbells in each hand while performing the exercise.

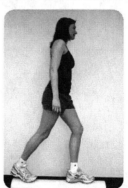

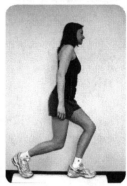

Starting position   Ending position

Turn and Lunge — quadriceps, with emphasis on the vastus medialis

Positioning   Stand with feet together.

Execution   Bring the right foot back while turning the body to the right. Shift the weight to the right leg while allowing left knee to bend slightly.

Client reminders   Do not allow the knees to pass over the toes. Keep the left foot stationary. Repeat on the other side.

Modifications   Hold dumbbells in each hand while performing the exercise.

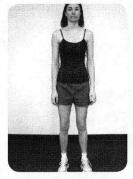 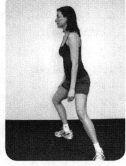

Starting position   Ending position

Crossovers — quadriceps

Positioning   Stand with feet shoulder-width apart.

Execution   Cross the right foot in front of the left and bend both knees. Allow the left heel to come up off the floor.

Client reminders   Keep the left foot stationary. Repeat on the other side.

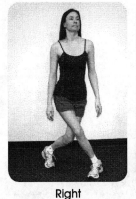 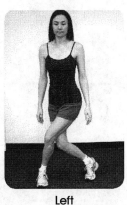

Right   Left

Side Lunge with Toe Touch — quadriceps

Positioning   Stand with feet together.

Execution   Take a large step to the side with the left foot and bend the right knee. Allow the other knee to bend. Reach toward the toes with both hands.

Client reminders   Do not allow the knees to pass over the toes. Keep the left foot stationary. Contract the abdominals and keep the back flat. Repeat on the other side.

Modifications   Hold dumbbells in each hand while performing the exercise.

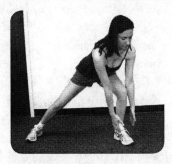

Side Squats with Ball   quadriceps

Positioning   Lean one side of the trunk into a stability ball that is against a wall. Pick up the foot that is farthest from the wall.
Execution   Slowly bend the knee and then return to the starting position.
Client reminders   Do not allow the knee to pass over the toes. Repeat on the other side.
Modifications
- Use different size stability balls.
- Pick up the foot that is closest to the wall and cross it behind the other. Performing side squats in this position will emphasize the vastus medialis of the supporting leg.

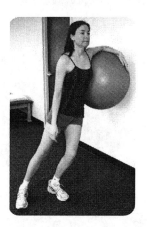
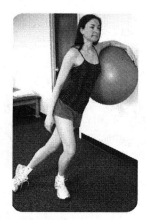

Modification to emphasize vastus medialis

Backward Lunge with Rotation   quadriceps and hamstrings

Positioning   Stand with feet together holding a medicine ball with both hands at shoulder height.
Execution   Step back with the right foot into a lunge position. Rotate the trunk and bring the ball to the right side. Bring the ball back in front of the body before bringing the feet back together.
Client reminders   Keep the weight shifted onto the back leg and rotate the ball to the same side as the back leg. Keep the ball elevated at shoulder height. Repeat on the other side.
Note   Do not perform this exercise if the client experiences back pain.

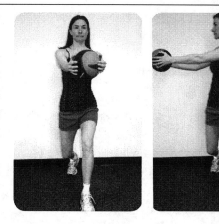

Deadlifts   hamstrings

Positioning   Stand with feet shoulder-width apart

Execution   Lean forward at the waist, allowing the hands to reach toward the floor. Keep the back flat and contract the abdominals while moving to an upright position. Return to the starting position.

Client reminders   Do not round the back and keep the abdominals contracted.

Modifications   Hold dumbbells or a barbell while performing this exercise.

Note   Do not perform this exercise if the client experiences back pain.

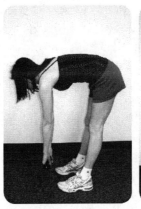 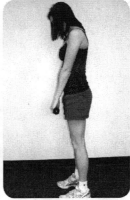

Starting position   Ending position

Squat Sits   quadriceps and hamstrings

Positioning   Stand in front of a chair or elevated box with feet shoulder-width apart.

Execution   Bend both knees and slowly lower the body. Stop the movement just before the buttocks contact the chair or box.

Client reminders   Do not allow the knees to pass over the toes. Keep the back flat and contract the abdominals.

Modifications   Decrease the height of the chair or box. Hold dumbbells or a barbell while performing this exercise.

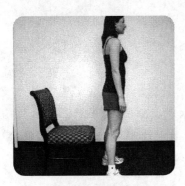 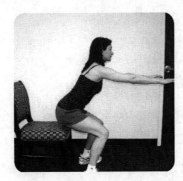

Starting position   Ending position

Single-Leg Swimmers   quadriceps and hamstrings

Positioning   In each hand, grasp the ends of a resistance band that is securely tied to an object at waist height. Pick up one foot and slightly bend the other knee. Lean the trunk forward so it is almost parallel to the floor and allow the other leg to move posteriorly.

Execution   Alternately pull the resistance band backward on each side. Repeat 10–20 times on each arm before lowering the other foot to the floor.

Client reminders   Keep the knee slightly bent and the body weight centered over the stationary leg. Keep the back straight and contract the abdominals. Repeat on the other side.

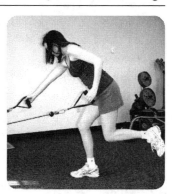

Modifications

- Increase the resistance of the band or place more tension on the band prior to initiating movement.
- Pull only one end of the resistive band back.
- Pull both ends of the resistive band back at the same time.

Uneven Single-Leg Squat and Hold   quadriceps and hamstrings

Positioning   Stand on an uneven surface (foam pad, air-filled cushion, pillow).

Execution   Pick one foot up and slightly bend the other knee. Hold this position without losing balance.

Client reminders   Try not to let the other foot touch the floor. Keep the knee slightly bent and the body weight centered over the stationary leg. Keep your back straight and contract the abdominals. Repeat on the other side.

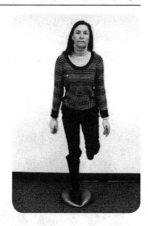

Modifications

- Increase the amount of time in the squatting position.
- Throw the client a ball while he or she attempts to maintain balance.
- Instruct the client to trace the letters of the alphabet with the elevated foot.
- Perform the exercise without shoes.

Single-Leg Squat and Reach   quadriceps and hamstrings

Positioning   Stand in front of an object that is 12–18 inches away and approximately 12 inches off the ground (e.g., a cone). Pick the left foot off the floor.

Execution   Bend the right knee and reach for the top of the object with the left hand. As the trunk leans forward, allow the left leg to move posteriorly. Return to the starting position.

Client reminders   The trunk and the left leg move at the same time with the hips acting as a fulcrum. Do not allow the knee to pass over the toes. Keep the back flat and contract the abdominals. Repeat on the other side.

Modifications   Place the object at different angles in front of the body to work on different planes of movement.

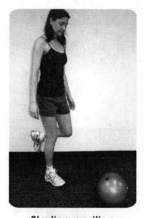
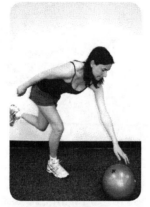

Starting position   Ending position

Single-Leg Pick-Up   quadriceps and hamstrings

Positioning   Place 10 small, hand-held objects in a semi-circle on the floor approximately 12–18 inches in front of the feet. Lift one foot off the floor.

Execution   Slowly bend the knee and pick up the objects on the floor. Repeat until all the objects are picked up.

Client reminders   Do not allow the knee to pass over the toes. Keep the back flat and contract the abdominals. Repeat on the other side.

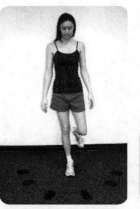
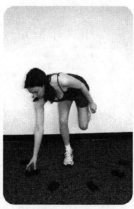

Starting position   Ending position

Flexibility Exercises

Flexibility exercises are important for maintaining balance of the muscles surrounding the knee joint. All clients should perform flexibility exercises of both the quadriceps and hamstring muscle groups as part of their comprehensive fitness routine. Remind the client to count slowly for 20 or 30 seconds and repeat the exercise 3 to 5 times on each leg.

Supine Hamstrings Stretch   hamstrings

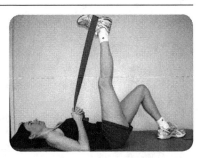

Positioning   Lie on your back.
Execution   Lift the straightened leg toward the ceiling and hold on to the back of the thigh. Hold for 20-30 seconds.
Client reminder   Keep the knee as straight as possible. Do not allow the back to arch. Repeat on the other side.
Modification   Place a towel or strap around the arch of the foot to assist the stretch.

Standing Hamstrings Stretch   hamstrings

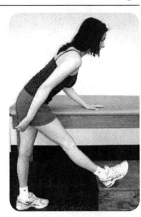

Positioning   Standing, prop one heel on a stool or step.
Execution   Lean forward at the waist with the trunk straight. Hold for 20–30 seconds.
Client reminder   Keep the back flat and the knee straight. Do not round the back and keep the abdominals contracted. Repeat on the other side.
Common errors   Rounding the back. Putting the foot flat on the stool.

Heel-to-Buttocks Stretch

quadriceps

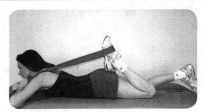

Positioning   Lie prone on a mat.

Execution   With a towel or strap wrapped around the foot or ankle of one leg, bend the knee and pull the foot toward the buttocks. Hold for 20–30 seconds.

Client reminder   Keep both hips on the mat. Repeat on the other side.

Common error   Twisting away from the side that is stretched.

Note   Do not perform if client has increased pain with knee flexion.

Standing Quadriceps Stretch

quadriceps

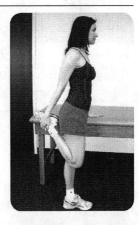

Positioning   While standing, bend one knee and grasp the ankle behind the body.

Execution   Gently pull the foot toward the buttocks. Keep both thighs parallel to one another. Hold for 20–30 seconds. Use support for balance if needed.

Client reminders   Stand up straight and do not lean forward. Repeat on the other side.

Note   Do not perform if client has increased pain with knee flexion.

Gastrocnemius Stretch

gastrocnemius

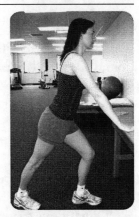

Positioning   Standing, place both hands against a wall or chair for support and place one foot behind the other.

Execution   Bend the front knee toward the wall and keep the back knee straight. Hold for 20–30 seconds.

Client reminder   Press the back heel into the floor. Repeat on the other side.

Common errors   Feet too far apart. Allowing the back heel to lift off the floor.

Gastrocnemius Stretch on Step

gastrocnemius

Positioning Stand on a stool or step. A support can be used for balance. Bring one heel off the edge of the step.

Execution Drop the heel below the step, keeping the knee straight. Slightly bend the opposite knee. Hold for 20–30 seconds.

Client reminders Stand up straight. Repeat on the other side.

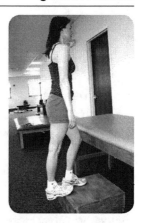

Standing Iliotibial Band Stretch

iliotibial band

Positioning Standing with the right hip toward a wall, cross the left foot in front of the right foot and place the right hand or elbow on the wall for support.

Execution Gently lean the right hip toward the wall. A stretch should be felt on the outside of the right leg and hip area. Hold for 20–30 seconds.

Client reminders Do not lean the trunk forward or sidebend excessively. Keep the abdominals contracted. Do not allow the entire body to lean toward the wall. Repeat on the other side.

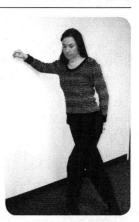

Foam Roller Iliotibial Band Stretch

iliotibial band

Positioning Lie with the right hip on top of a full-round foam roller perpendicular to the body. Place the sole of the left foot on the ground in front of or behind the straightened right leg. The body weight can be supported by the right hand or elbow.

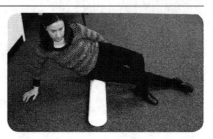

Execution Gently roll the foam roller up and down the length of the outer thigh to the level of the knee for 1–2 minutes. Repeat on the other side.

Client reminders Keep the abdominals contract-ed. Discontinue exercise if client experiences pain in the leg or the back.

Study Questions

Complete the following questions. The answer key is on page 109.

1. True or false: Closed kinetic chain exercises are those in which the foot is not in contact with a solid surface.

2. Name two examples of open kinetic chain exercises and two examples of closed kinetic chain exercises.

   Open kinetic chain exercise:

   (1) _____

   (2) _____

   Closed kinetic chain exercise:

   (1) _____

   (2) _____

3. List two beginner exercises that emphasize the vastus medialis:

   (1) _____

   (2) _____

4. True or false: One way in which to modify the Step-Up exercise is to increase the height of the step.

5. List three intermediate exercises that emphasize the hamstrings.

   (1) _____

   (2) _____

   (3) _____

6. True or false: To emphasize the vastus medialis during the Wall Squats, turn the toes out to a 45-degree angle.

Chapter **5**

Case Studies

This chapter outlines two case studies that are typically seen by fitness professionals. Information is given regarding the client's history, the results of the assessment, and the goals of the knee program. A sample exercise routine and an appropriate progression of the exercises are also presented.

History of ACL Reconstruction Surgery

History

A 21-year-old female client comes to the facility during the summer break between her junior and senior years in college. She is hoping to try out for the college soccer team in the fall and would like help with a conditioning and strengthening routine. During the school year she works out at the gym about three times a week. She had an ACL reconstruction (bone-patellar-bone autograft) of her right knee during her freshman year in high school. Her last appointment with the surgeon was four years ago, and at that time she was cleared to participate in all forms of activities. The client has no other pertinent medical history.

Assessment

The assessment reveals decreased flexibility of her hamstrings bilaterally. Her quadriceps flexibility is slightly decreased on the right side, and her strength is normal bilaterally. She has some forward flexion of her trunk when she performs the Single-Leg Stability test on the right. She does not experience any pain during the testing.

Goals

The client will work toward achieving the following goals within one to two months:
- Improve the flexibility of the hamstrings and quadriceps.
- Increase single-leg stability, especially on the right side.
- Improve knee strength.
- Improve cardiovascular fitness in preparation for soccer tryouts.
- Become educated on the PEP Program for ACL injury prevention.

Exercise Routine

This exercise routine should be performed at least three to four times per week. Begin the workout session with cardiovascular conditioning. The most appropriate mode of exercise would be jogging or running on the treadmill in preparation for soccer. Depending on her cardiovascular conditioning level, she should perform at least 20 minutes of activity and increase the time and speed as tolerated.

Flexibility exercises for her quadriceps and hamstrings should be performed next, followed by strengthening for the knees. The following are some appropriate exercises to address the client's knee flexibility, strength, and stability. The client will most likely be challenged by the intermediate and advanced exercises since she has already been training at the gym on a regular basis. Closed kinetic chain exercises will place the client in functional positions without increasing the shear forces on the right knee.

Flexibility exercises
- Standing Hamstrings Stretch
- Standing Quadriceps Stretch
- Standing Gastrocnemius Stretch on Step

Strengthening exercises
- Wall Squats
- Resistance Band Leg Pulls
- Step Dips
- Stool Pulls
- Hamstrings Curls on Ball
- Turn and Lunge
- Squat Sits
- Crossovers
- Resistance Band Single-Leg Squats

- Single-Leg Swimmers
- Single-Leg Pick-Up
- Single-Leg Squat and Reach

The client would also benefit from strengthening exercises for the hip and ankle. Examples of these exercises are not included in the scope of this book.

Instruction in the PEP program for ACL injury prevention would also be appropriate for this client. She may be interested to learn that athletes who had a history of ACL injury and participated in the PEP program were significantly less likely to suffer another ACL injury compared with athletes who did not perform the PEP program (Gilchrist et al. 2008). If there is adequate room in the facility, the client may perform this warm-up routine before beginning the training session.

Exercise Progression

In general, these exercises should progress as follows:

- Start with 2 sets of 10 repetitions and progress to 3 sets of 10.
- Increase the resistance of the band once 3 sets of 10 become easier for the client to complete. If necessary, decrease the repetitions when the resistance is increased.
- Progress the Wall Squats to Single-Leg Wall Squats.
- Monitor the client's heart rate and perceived exertion during the course of the workout.

Previous Knee Injury

History

A 65-year-old female asks to work with a fitness professional at your facility because she feels a little "weak in her knees" and wants to improve her leg strength. She retired three years ago from a retail sales position that required her to stand for almost eight hours a day. Since this time, she has not been very active, except for playing with her grandchildren. She tells you that she sometimes has difficulty getting out of chairs and needs to take the elevator to her third floor apartment instead of taking the stairs, but she does not currently complain of any pain in the knees.

About six months ago, she tripped and fell on to her right knee. At that time she had increased pain on the inside of her knee and some minor swelling. An MRI was negative for ligament or meniscal tears, and x-rays of the knee showed mild degenerative changes. The doctor diagnosed her with a Grade 1 medial collateral ligament sprain. During a recent doctor's appointment, her physician recommended that she start an exercise program, so she is looking for assistance in developing a personalized workout routine.

Assessment

The assessment reveals that the client has decreased flexibility in both her hamstrings and quadriceps. Her quadriceps strength is diminished on both sides; however, the right side is weaker than the left. She is unable to stand on one foot to complete the Single-Leg Stability test. She did not have any pain during the testing. The left leg's muscle girth is one-quarter inch larger than the right side.

Goals

The client will work toward achieving the following goals within two to three months:
- Increase the flexibility of the quadriceps and hamstrings.
- Increase knee strength, especially the quadriceps, so that the client is able to get out of a chair without difficulty and also climb the stairs to her third floor apartment as desired.
- Increase single-leg balance.
- Increase cardiovascular fitness so that she can play with her grandchildren.

Exercise Routine

This exercise routine should be performed three times per week. Begin the workout session with cardiovascular conditioning. The client can use either the recumbent bike or the treadmill to increase the circulation and warm up the muscles. She should perform 10–20 minutes of activity depending on the client's current cardiovascular conditioning.

Flexibility exercises for her quadriceps and hamstrings should be performed first:
- Supine Hamstrings Stretch
- Heel-to-Buttocks Stretch
- Gastrocnemius Stretch

Exercises to improve her knee strength and stability should follow her flexibility training. The client would benefit from any of the beginner exercises, such as:
- Resistance Band Quadriceps Push
- Pillow Squeeze
- Straight-Leg Lift
- Leg Kick-Out
- Standing Hamstrings Curl

She may also be able to perform some of the intermediate exercises.

- Standing Knee Extension with Resistance Band
- Resistance Band Leg Pulls
- Hamstrings Curl with Resistance Band
- Wall Squats
- Step-Ups
- Forward and Backward Lunges

Eventually the client may be able to progress to some of the advanced exercises, such as:

- Step Dips
- Turn and Lunge
- Squat Sits
- Single-Leg Wall Squats

Exercise Progression

In general, these exercises should progress as follows:

- Start with 2 sets of 10 repetitions and progress to 3 sets of 10.
- Increase the resistance of the band once 3 sets of 10 become easier for the client to complete. If necessary, decrease the repetitions when the resistance is increased.
- Increase the height of the steps
- Monitor the client's heart rate and perceived exertion during the course of the workout.

Appendix: PEP Program

Reprinted with permission from "The PEP Program," Santa Monica Orthopaedic and Sports Research Foundation: ACL Prevention Program.

The field should be set up 10 minutes prior to the warm-up to allow for easy transition between the activities. The program takes approximately 15 to 20 minutes to complete. The proper amount of time to spend on each activity is listed next to the individual exercise, which will serve as a guideline in order to conduct the warm-up in a time-efficient manner.

Sample Field Set-up

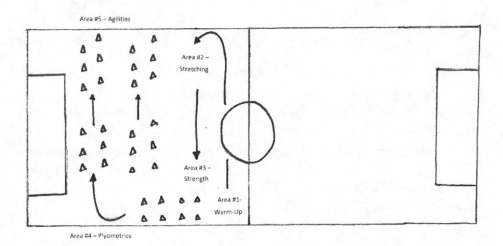

Warm-Up

Warming up and cooling down are crucial parts of a training program. The purpose of the warm-up section is to allow the athlete to prepare for activity. By warming up your muscles first, you greatly reduce the risk of injury.

1. JOG-LINE-TO-LINE (CONE-TO-CONE):

Elapsed time   0–0.5 minute

Purpose   Allows the athletes to slowly prepare themselves for the training session while minimizing the risk of injury. Educate athletes on good running technique: keep the hip/knee/ankle in straight alignment without the knee caving in or the feet whipping out to the sides.

Instruction   Complete a slow jog from near to far sideline.

2. SHUTTLE RUN (SIDE-TO-SIDE)

Elapsed time   0.5–1 minute

Purpose   To engage hip muscles (inner and outer thigh). This exercise promotes increased speed and discourages inward caving of the knee joint.

Instruction   Start in an athletic stance with a slight bend at the knee. Leading with the right foot, sidestep while pushing off with the left foot (back leg). When you drive off with the back leg, be sure the hip/knee/ankle are in a straight line. Switch sides at half field.

3. BACKWARD RUNNING

Elapsed time   1–1.5 minutes

Purpose   Continued warm-up; engage hip extensors/hamstrings. Make sure the athlete lands on the toes. Be sure to watch for locking of the knee joint. As the athlete brings the foot back, make sure she maintains a slight bend in the knee.

Instruction   Run backward from sideline to sideline. Land on your toes without snapping the knee back. Stay on your toes and keep the knees slightly bent at all times.

Stretching

It is important to incorporate a short warm-up prior to stretching. Never stretch a cold muscle. By performing the exercises outlined here, the athlete can improve and maintain range of motion, reduce stiffness in joints, reduce postexercise soreness, reduce the risk of injury, and improve overall mobility and performance.

- Do a large muscle warm-up, such as brisk walking, for 5–10 minutes before stretching.
- Don't bounce or jerk when you stretch. Gently stretch to a point of tension and hold.
- Hold the stretch for 30 seconds. Concentrate on lengthening the muscles when you're stretching.
- Breathe normally. Don't hold your breath.

1. CALF STRETCH: 30 SECONDS X 2 REPETITIONS

Elapsed time	1.5–2.5 minutes
Purpose	To stretch the calf muscle of the lower leg.
Instruction	Stand while leading with your right leg. Bend forward at the waist and place your hands on the ground (V formation). Keep your right knee slightly bent and your left leg straight. Make sure your left foot is flat on the ground. Do not bounce during the stretch. Hold for 30 seconds. Switch sides and repeat.

2. QUADRICEPS STRETCH: 30 SECONDS X 2 REPETITIONS

Elapsed time	2.5–3.5 minutes
Purpose	To stretch the quadricep muscles of the front of the thigh.
Instruction	Place your left hand on your partner's left shoulder. Reach back with your right hand and grab the front of your right ankle. Bring your heel to your buttock, making sure your knee is pointed down toward the ground. Keep your right leg close to your left leg. Don't allow your knee to wing out to the side, and do not bend at the waist. Hold for 30 seconds and switch sides.

3. FIGURE-FOUR HAMSTRING STRETCH: 30 SECONDS X 2 REPETITIONS

Elapsed time   3.5–4.5 minutes

Purpose   To stretch the hamstring muscles of the back of the thigh.

Instruction   Sit on the ground with your right leg extended out in front of you. Bend your left knee and rest the bottom of your foot on your right inner thigh. With a straight back, try to bring your chest toward your knee. Do not round your back. If you can, reach down toward your toes and pull them up toward your head. Do not bounce. Hold for 30 seconds and repeat with the other leg.

4. INNER THIGH STRETCH: 20 SECONDS X 2 REPETITIONS

Elapsed time   4.5–5.5 minutes

Purpose   To elongate the muscle of the inner thigh (adductor group).

Instruction   Remain seated on the ground. Spread your legs apart evenly. Slowly lower yourself to the center with a straight back. You want to feel a stretch in the inner thigh. Now reach toward the right with the right arm. Bring your left arm overhead and stretch over to the right. Hold the stretch and repeat on the opposite side.

5. HIP FLEXOR STRETCH: 30 SECONDS X 2 REPETITIONS

Elapsed time   5.5 – 6.5 minutes

Purpose   To elongate the hip flexors of the front of the thigh.

Instruction   Lunge forward leading with your right leg. Drop your left knee down to the ground. Placing your hands on top of your right thigh, lean forward with your hips. The hips should be square with your shoulders. If possible, maintain your balance and lift back for the left ankle and pull your heel to your buttocks. Hold for 30 seconds and repeat on the other side.

Strengthening

This portion of the program focuses on increasing leg strength to improve knee joint stability. Technique is everything--close attention must be paid to the performance of these exercises in order to avoid injury.

1. WALKING LUNGES: 3 SETS X 10 REPETITIONS

Elapsed time   6.5–7.5 minutes

Purpose   To strengthen the quadricep muscles.

Instruction   Lunge forward while leading with your right leg. Push off with your right leg and lunge forward with your left leg. Drop the knee straight down. Make sure you keep your front knee over your ankle. Control the motion and try to avoid your front knee from caving inward. Note: If you cannot see your toes on your leading leg, you are doing the exercise incorrectly.

2. RUSSIAN HAMSTRING: 3 SETS X 10 REPETITIONS

Elapsed time   7.5–8.5 minutes

Purpose   To strengthen the hamstring muscles.

Instruction   Kneel on the ground with your hands at your side. Have a partner hold your legs firmly at the ankles. With a straight back, lean forward leading with your hips. Your knee, hip, and shoulder should be in a straight line as you lean toward the ground. Do not bend at the waist. You should feel the hamstrings in the back of your thigh working.

3. SINGLE-TOE RAISES: 30 REPS X 2 REPETITIONS

Elapsed time   8.5–9.5 minutes

Purpose   To strengthen the calf muscle and increase balance.

Instruction   Stand up with your arms at your side. Bend the left knee and maintain balance. Slowly rise up on your right toes with good balance. You may hold your arms out ahead. Slowly repeat 30 times and switch to the other side. As you get stronger, you may need to add additional repetitions to this exercise to continue its strengthening effect.

Plyometrics

These exercises are explosive and help to build power, strength, and speed. The most important element when considering performance technique is the landing. It must be soft! When landing from a jump, the athlete needs to softly accept the weight on the balls of the feet, slowly rolling back onto the heels with bent knees and even hips. These exercises are basic; however, it is crucial to perform them correctly. Please take the time to ensure safe and correct performance of these exercises.

1. LATERAL HOPS OVER CONE: 20 REPETITIONS

Elapsed time   9.5–10 minutes

Purpose   To increase power and strength while emphasizing neuromuscular control.

Instruction   Stand with a 6" cone to your left. Hop to the left over the cone, softly landing on the balls of your feet and with bent knees. Repeat this exercise hopping to the right.

2. FORWARD/BACKWARD HOPS OVER CONE: 20 REPETITIONS

Elapsed time   10–10.5 minutes

Purpose   To increase power and strength while emphasizing neuromuscular control.

Instruction   Hop over the cone, softly landing on the balls of your feet and with bent knees. Now, hop backward over the cone using the same landing technique. Be careful not to snap your knee back to straighten it. You want to maintain a slight bend in the knees throughout the exercise.

3. SINGLE-LEG HOPS OVER CONE: 20 REPETITIONS

Elapsed time   10.5–11 minutes

Purpose   To increase power and strength while emphasizing neuromuscular control.

Instruction   Hop over the cone, landing on one leg on the ball of the foot and with bent knee. Now, hop backward over the cone, using the same landing technique. Be careful not to snap your knee back to straighten it. Maintain a slight bend in the knees throughout the exercise. Repeat for 20 repetitions. Now, stand on the left leg and repeat the exercise. Increase the number of repetitions as needed.

4. VERTICAL JUMPS WITH HEADERS: 20 REPETITIONS

Elapsed time	11–11.5 minutes
Purpose	To increase the height of the athlete's vertical jump.
Instruction	Stand forward with your hands at your side. Slightly bend the knees and push off, jumping straight up. Remember, the proper landing technique: accept the weight on the ball of your foot with a slight bend in the knees. Repeat 20 times and switch sides.

5. SCISSORS JUMP: 20 REPETITIONS

Elapsed time	11.5–12 minutes
Purpose	To increase the power and strength of the vertical jump.
Instruction	Lunge forward, leading with your right leg. Keep your knee over your ankle. Now, push off with your right foot and propel your left leg forward into a lunge position. Be sure your knee does not cave in or out. It should be stable and directly over the ankle. Remember, the proper landing technique: accept the weight on the ball of your foot with a slight bend in the knees. Repeat 20 times.

Agilities

1. SHUTTLE RUN WITH FORWARD/BACKWARD RUNNING

Elapsed time	12–13 minutes
Purpose	To increase the dynamic stability of the ankle/knee/hip complex.
Instruction	Starting at the first cone, sprint forward to the second cone, run backward to the third cone, sprint forward to the fourth cone, and so on.

2. DIAGONAL RUNS: 3 PASSES

Elapsed time	13–14 minutes
Purpose	To encourage proper technique and improve stabilization of the outside planted foot to deter the position from occurring.
Instruction	Face forward and run to the first cone on the left. Pivot off the left foot and run to the second one. Now pivot off the right leg and continue on to the third cone. Make sure the outside leg does not cave in. Keep a slight bend in the knees and make sure the leading knee stays over the ankle joint.

3. BOUNDING RUN: 44 YARDS

Elapsed time   14–15 minutes

Purpose   To increase hip flexion strength and increase power and speed.

Instruction   Starting on the near sideline, run to the far side with knees up toward chest. Bring your knees up high. Land on the ball of your foot with a slight bend in the knees and even hips. Increase the distance as this exercise gets easier.

Alternative Exercises: Warm-Down and Cool-Down

We all know how imperative a cool-down is. Please don't allow clients to skip it. A cool-down allows the muscles that have been worked hard throughout the training session to elongate and it deters the onset of muscle soreness. Emphasize the importance of adequate fluid intake (ideally, water). Athletes should have a water bottle by their side during the cool-down. The cool-down should take approximately 10 minutes. Begin with a slow jog to allow the heart rate to come down before stretching. The slow jog should be followed by light strength training exercises (see below). Following the exercise stretch the hamstrings, calves, inner thighs, quadriceps, and low back (all of these are explained in the protocol). In addition to these basic stretches, some additional stretches to target three muscle groups are suggested.

Cool-Down

1. BRIDGING WITH ALTERNATING HIP FLEXION: 30 REPETITIONS

Purpose   To strengthen the outer hip muscles (hip abductors, flexors) and buttocks.

Instruction   Lie on the ground with your knees bent and with feet on the ground. Raise your buttocks up off the ground and squeeze. Now, lift your right foot off the ground, making sure your right hip does not dip down. Lower your right foot and lift your left foot, making sure your left hip does not dip down. Repeat 30 times on each side. As you get stronger, you will place your feet on a ball to perform the exercise.

2. ABDOMINAL CRUNCHES: 30 REPS X 2 REPETITIONS

Purpose   To strengthen the abdominals (rectus abdominus, obliques).

Instruction   Lie on the ground with your knees bent. Place your hands behind your head with your elbows wide. Support your neck lightly with your fingers. Take a deep breath in and slowly contract your abdominal muscles as you exhale. Repeat 30 times. Drop your legs off to the right side. Slowly crunch up with your elbows out wide. You should feel your oblique muscles working on the other side of your waist. Repeat 30 times and switch to the other side.

3. SINGLE AND DOUBLE KNEE-TO-CHEST: (SUPINE) 30 SECONDS X 2 REPETITIONS

Purpose   To elongate the low back muscles.

Instruction   Lie on your back. Bring your right knee toward your chest and hug firmly. Keep your left leg straight in front of you. You should feel a stretch along your low back and down to your buttocks. Hold the stretch for 30 seconds and switch sides. Now bring both knees to your chest. If you feel any pain in the low back, discontinue the stretch and inform your coach/trainer.

4. FIGURE-FOUR PIRIFORMIS STRETCH (SUPINE): 30 SECONDS X 2 REPETITIONS

Purpose   To elongate the rotators of the hip.

Instruction   Lie on your back and bend both your knees. Fold your left ankle over your right knee. Place your hands behind your right thigh and pull your right knee to your chest. You should feel a good stretch in the left gluteals region and the side of the thigh. Hold for 30 seconds and repeat on the other side. If you experience any low back pain with this stretch, slowly lower your legs and let your coach/trainer know.

5. SEATED BUTTERFLY STRETCH: 30 SECONDS X 2 REPETITIONS

Purpose   To elongate the inner thigh muscles (adductors).

Instruction   In a seated position, bring your feet in toward the groin so that the soles of your feet are touching. Gently place your elbows on your knees and slowly push down. You should feel a good stretch of the inner thigh. Hold for 30 seconds and repeat 2–3 times.

Warm-Up

The following are the replacement exercises for the Alternative Warm-Up Program. These exercises can be performed instead of the original program for variety, but they were not part of the original scientific study that demonstrated a decrease in female ACL injury rates.

1. LAP AROUND THE FIELD: 2–3 LAPS

Purpose   To increase heart rate.

Instruction   Slowly jog around the perimeter of the field for 2–3 laps to increase heart rate and prepare for the day's training session.

2. BACKWARD RUNNING WITH HEEL SLAP: 20–40 YARDS

Purpose   To increase coordination, increase heart rate, and engage hamstrings.

Instruction   Run backward from sideline to sideline. As you bring your heel toward your buttock, strike the side of your ankle with your hand. Repeat on opposite side. Remember proper landing technique: land on your toes with slight knee and hip flexion (bending).

Stretching

1. Standing Calf Stretch with Straight Knee and Bent Knee: 30–60 seconds

Purpose   To stretch the gastrocnemius and soleus of the lower extremity.

Instruction   Stand in a lunge position with the right leg forward and the left leg back. Keep the left knee straight and the left heel on the ground. The right knee should be bent 90 degrees. Hold the stretch for 30–60 seconds. Slightly bend the left leg (back leg) and hold for 30–60 seconds. Repeat on the opposite side.

2. SIDELYING QUADRICEPS STRETCH: 30–60 SECONDS

Purpose   To stretch the quadricep muscles.

Instruction   Lie on your left side in a straight line: shoulder, hip, knee, and ankles should be aligned. Reach back for your right ankle, grab hold of it, and pull your right hip backward. Feel the stretch across the front of the right thigh. Hold for 30–60 seconds and repeat on the opposite side.

3. SIDELYING QUADRICEPS STRETCH WITH CONTRALATERAL HIP FLEXION WITH HEEL GRAB: 30–60 SECONDS

Purpose   To stretch the hip flexor muscles.

Instruction   Lie on your left side in a straight line: shoulder, hip, knee, and ankles should be aligned. Bend the left hip and knee to 90 degrees (right-angle position). Reach back for your right ankle and pull the right leg backward. Feel the stretch along the junction of the hip and thigh. Hold for 30–60 seconds and repeat on the opposite side.

4. BUTTERFLY STRETCH: 30–60 SECONDS

Purpose   To stretch the adductor (inner thigh).

Instruction   In a seated position, bend your knees and bring your feet toward your groin with the soles of your feet together. Attempt to get the outside of your knee to the ground. You may use your elbows to push on the inside of the knee. Hold for 30–60 seconds.

5. PRETZEL STRETCH (SI JOINT): 30–60 SECONDS

Purpose   To stretch the deep hip rotators and gluteals.

Instruction   Lie on your back, folding your right knee directly over the left knee. Pull your knees to chest and feel the stretch on the right side of your hip and leg. Hold for 30–60 seconds and repeat with the opposite leg.

6. PRONE CAT STRETCH WITH LATERAL STRETCH: 30–60 SECONDS

Purpose   To stretch the low back and transverse muscles.

Instruction   From a hands-and-knees position, sit back onto your heels with arms stretched in front of you as far as possible. Hold stretch for 30 seconds. Now, side bend to the right and reach your arms ahead of you. You should feel a good stretch on the left side. Hold the stretch for 30 seconds and repeat this stretch to the left.

Strengthening

1. SINGLE-LEG SQUAT: 3 SETS OF 10 REPETITIONS

Purpose To strengthen the quadriceps and improve balance.

Instruction Stand with feet together. Bend right hip/knee to approximately 90 degrees. With all of your weight on the left leg (stance leg), squat down on the left leg while maintaining your balance. The goal is to achieve 90 degrees of knee flexion (bend) on the stance leg but begin the exercise in a comfortable range. Perform a set and repeat on the opposite leg.

2. CROSSOVER LUNGES: 20 YARDS

Purpose To increase strength of the lower extremity and improve coordination.

Instruction Similar to walking lunges. Lunge forward leading with your right leg; however, cross your right leg over the midline. Bend your right knee to 60–90 degrees (as tolerated). Now bring the left leg across the right. Lunge forward, alternating legs for 20 yards. You may increase the yardage as you gain strength.

3. BRIDGING ON BALL (KNEE-TO-CHEST): 3 SETS OF 10 REPETITIONS

Purpose To strengthen the hamstrings and hips.

Instruction Lying on your back with knees bent, place both feet on top of a soccer ball. Lift your hips off ground so that your shoulders, hips, and knees are in a straight line. Slowly straighten knees and then bring your knees to the chest (without lowering hips).

4. TOE TOUCH ON BALL (QUICK FEET): 3 SETS OF 1-MINUTE DURATION

Purpose To increase calf strength and coordination.

Instruction Standing with the ball slightly ahead of you, place your toe on top of the ball (without moving it) and quickly switch feet. Repeat exercise for 1 minute and rest.

5. HIP BAND WALKING (A/P AND LATERAL): 20 YARDS

Purpose   To increase lower extremity and trunk strength and build dynamic stability.

Instruction   Resistance band needed for this exercise. Place band around your ankles. Face forward and repeat walking lunge exercise using resistance band. Remember to keep your knee over the ankle to prevent excessive pressure on the knee. Now, step out with the right leg to the side and squat down, keeping the knee over the ankle joint. Bring your left leg to the right and repeat this for a distance of 20 yards. Repeat the exercise leading with the left leg. You can increase yardage as you get stronger.

Plyometrics

1. DIAGONAL PLYOMETRICS: 20 REPETITIONS

Purpose   To increase power, strength, and coordination of the lower extremity.

Instruction   Stand with a small flat cone (2" in height) in front of you to your right. Hop over the cone in a diagonal fashion, landing on the balls of your feet while bending at the hips and knees. Now, hop backward and to the left over the cone to return to your starting position. Repeat 20 times and then step to the left and repeat the exercise in the opposite diagonal.

2. SUCCESSIVE PLYOMETRIC JUMPS WITH SPRINT (8–10 CONES WITH 20-YARD SPRINT): 3 REPETITIONS

Purpose   To increase power and strength.

Instruction   Place 8-10 cones in a straight line approximately 18 - 24" apart. Hop over each cone quickly with proper landing technique: on your toes with bent hips and bent knees. After the last cone, sprint for 20 yards and slowly jog to the starting point.

3. JUMP AND TUCK: 20 REPETITIONS FOR 1-3 SETS (STRENGTH DEPENDENT)

Purpose   To increase hip strength and power.

Instruction   Jump up bringing your knees toward your chest (tucked position). Land on your toes with the hips and knees bent (flexion), and quickly repeat the exercise. Increase the number of repetitions and sets as you gain strength.

Agilities

1. STAR EXERCISE: 3 REPETITIONS

Purpose   To increase balance (proprioception) and coordination.

Instruction   Place five cones in a circular fashion and stand in the center of the cones. Stand on your right foot with a slightly bent knee. Reach for each cone while maintaining balance. To increase the difficulty of this exercise, close your eyes while you reach for each cone. Repeat the exercise for 1 minute then rest.

2. TWO-CONE TWIST AND REACH: 30 REPETITIONS

Purpose   To increase hip strength and balance.

Instruction   Place two cones at a 45-degree angle from your hip (2 o'clock and 10 o'clock position). Stand on your right foot with your knee slightly bent. Reach for the left cone with the right hand. Then reach for the right cone with the left hand. Do this quickly while maintaining your balance on one leg. Repeat 30 times and switch legs.

3. QUICK FEET (LADDER OR CONES): 10 YARDS

Purpose   To increase reaction time and power.

Instruction   Using a plyometric ladder or cones placed ahead of you, quickly step through each rung of the ladder (cone), pushing off with the ball of your foot. Slowly jog back to the starting point and repeat.

4. JUGGLE WITH BALL AT FEET/KNEES

Purpose   To improve lower extremity coordination.

Instruction   Juggle a soccer ball at the feet and knees (alternating) for 1-minute duration. To increase difficulty, use one leg only, attempting to control the ball.

Additional Exercises

1. BRIDGING WITH HIP EXTENSION: 30 REPETITIONS

Purpose   To increase hip and trunk strength and improve balance.

Instruction   Lying on your back with knees bent, place both feet on top of a soccer ball. Lift your hips off the ground so that your shoulders, hips, and knees are in a straight line. Slowly lift one foot off the ball and straighten the knee without dipping the hip down. Return foot back to the ball and repeat on the opposite leg.

2. BALL TOSS WITH ABDOMINAL TOSS (PARTNER): 30 REPETITIONS

Purpose   To increase abdominal and trunk strength.

Instruction   Lie on your back with hips and knees bent. Have your partner toss a soccer ball to you. Catch the ball and bring your arms overhead. Now, catapult yourself by bringing your arms back toward your center as you perform an abdominal crunch and toss the ball to your partner. Wait for your partner to toss the ball again and repeat.

Summary

The PEP program has gained national attention and has been recognized by the American Physical Therapy Association (APTA), National Collegiate Athletic Association (NCAA), and the Centers for Disease Control and Prevention (CDC). In a September 2008 press release, the APTA urged "female athletes—particularly soccer players—to consider a new warm-up program [PEP Program] to help lower their growing risk of anterior cruciate ligament (ACL) injuries" (American Physical Therapy Association 2008). The APTA concurred with the results of the 2008 Gilchrist study, saying that "specialized stretching, strengthening, agility and jumping exercises could lower the overall ACL injury rate among female athletes" (American Physical Therapy Association 2008).

The CDC issued a press release in July 2008 about the PEP program stating: "The risk of potentially devastating tears to an important knee ligament may be reduced in female college soccer players by an alternative warm-up program that focuses on stretching, strengthening, and improving balance and movements. The program can be done without additional equipment or extensive training that other prevention programs may require" (Centers for Disease Control 2008).

Finally, sports organizations such as the NCAA have posted interactive videos on their websites about preventing ACL injuries in female athletes and the use of the PEP program. Colleges and high schools nationwide have also started using the PEP program in hopes of reducing the injury rate in their female athletes. A copy of the PEP program can be downloaded online and a DVD is available to order through the Santa Monica Orthopaedic Sports Medicine and Research Foundation's website: www.aclprevent.com.

Answer Keys

Chapter 1

1. True; p. 1
2. Increase; greater; p. 2
3. False; p. 2
4. True; pp. 2–3
5. (1) rectus femoris; (2) vastus medialis; (3) vastus lateralis; (4) vastus intermedius; p. 3
6. (1) biceps femoris; (2) semitendinosus; (3) semimembranosus; p. 4
7. False; p. 4
8. (1) anterior cruciate ligament; (2) posterior cruciate ligament; (3) medial collateral ligament; (4) lateral collateral ligament; pp. 5–6
9. False; p. 5
10. True; p. 6
11. (1) suprapatellar (quadriceps) bursa; (2) prepatellar bursa; (3) superficial infrapatellar bursa; (4) deep infrapatellar bursa; (5) popliteus bursa; (6) pes anserine bursa; (7) gastrocnemius bursa; (8) semimembranosus bursa; pp. 7–8

Chapter 2

1. (1) a blow to the knee from contact sports, a fall, or motor vehicle accident; (2) repeated stress or overuse; (3) sudden turning, pivoting, stopping, cutting from side to side; (4) awkward landings from jumping or falling during sports; (5) rapidly growing bones; (6) degeneration from aging; p. 11
2. False; p. 13

3. (1) muscle imbalance or weakness around the knee; (2) abnormal rotation of the hip or tibia; (3) altered angle between the femur and tibia; pp. 13–14

4. (1) Osgood-Schlatter disease; (2) osteochondritis dissecans; (3) chondromalacia patella; (4) patellofemoral syndrome; pp. 13–17

5. Boy's football and wrestling; girl's soccer and basketball; p. 19

6. Patellar tendonitis; p. 20

7. (1) changing direction rapidly; (2) stopping suddenly; (3) landing from a jump; (4) direct contact or collision; p. 21

8. Twisting, hyperextension, valgus; p. 21

9. True; p. 21

10. False; p. 23

11. (1) patellar tendon autograft; (2) hamstring tendon autograft; (3); allograft; p. 22

12. True; p. 23

13. Alignment, anatomic, hormones, joint, strength, weight, activation, recruitment; p. 24

14. True; p. 25

15. (1) avoid vulnerable positions; (2) increase flexibility; (3) increase strength; (4) include plyometric exercises into training program; (5) increase proprioception through agilities; pp. 25–26

16. True; p. 27

17. c: medial meniscus and the anterior cruciate ligament; p. 28

18. (1) degenerative; (2) longitudinal; (3) bucket-handle; (4) flap; (5) radial or transverse; pp. 29–30

19. False; p. 30

20. True; p. 31

Chapter 3

1. (1) Have you ever had surgery on the knee, and if so, when? (2) What specific type of surgery did you undergo? (3) If you had an ACL reconstruction, do you know what type of technique the surgeon used? (4) Have you ever been treated by a physical therapist for your knee? (5) Has your physician ever given you any specific restrictions? (e.g., running, cutting or pivoting activities) (6) When did you last see the orthopedic surgeon who

performed your surgery? (7) What is your occupation? (8) What type of activities or sports do you participate in? (9) Do any activities associated with your job or sports aggravate pain in your knee? p. 38

2. (1) identifying health conditions and risk factors that put your client at risk when participating in an exercise program or may necessitate referral to a healthcare professional; (2) assisting in the design of an appropriate exercise program; (3) identifying possible contraindicated activities; (4) fulfilling legal and insurance requirements for you or your facility; (5) encouraging and maintaining communication with the client's healthcare provider; p. 37

3. (1) heart rate; (2) perceived exertion; (3) pain scale; (4) physical observation; pp. 39–40

4. False; p. 43

5. False; p. 47

6. True; p. 47

7. Single-leg stability; p. 50

Chapter 4

1. False; p. 55

2. Open kinetic chain: (1) quadriceps push; (2) pillow squeeze; (3) straight leg lift; (4) straight leg lift with toe out; (5) leg kick out; (6) sidelying abduction; (7) sidelying adduction; (8) standing hamstring curl; (9) bridges on ball; (10) hamstring curls with resistance band; (11) resistance band leg pulls (active leg); (12) hamstring curl and kick; (13) hamstring curls on ball; pp. 57–72

   Closed kinetic chain: (1) standing knee extension with resisted band; (2) resistance band leg pulls (standing leg); (3) wall squats; (4) resistance band squats; (5) step-ups; (6) forward lunge; (7) lunge with back leg on ball; (8) backward lunge; (9) step dips; (10) lunge and lift; (11) single-leg wall squats; (12) resistance band single-leg squats; (13) resistance band lunge; (14) foam roller squats; (15) foam roller lunges; (16) turn and lunge; (17) crossovers; (18) side lunge with toe touch; (19) side squats with ball; (20) backward lunge with rotation; (21) deadlifts; (22) squat sits; (23) single-leg swimmers; (24) uneven single-leg squat and hold; (25) single-leg squat and reach; (26) single-leg pick-up; pp. 62–79

3. (1) pillow squeeze; (2) straight leg lift with toe out; (3) sidelying adduction; pp. 57–59

4. True; p. 66

5. (1) hamstring curls with resisted band; (2) resistance band leg pulls (extension); (3) stool pulls; (4) forward lunge; (5) hamstring curl and kick; (6) lunge with back leg on ball; pp. 62–69

6. True; p. 65

References

American Academy of Orthopaedic Surgeons. 2007. Common Knee Injuries. AAOS, http://orthoinfo.aaos.org/topic.cfm?topic=A00325 (accessed March 31, 2009).

———. 2007. Knee Ligament Injuries. AAOS, http://orthoinfo.aaos.org/topic.cfm?topic=A00349 (accessed March 1, 2009).

———. 2009. Total Knee Replacement. AAOS, http://orthoinfo.aaos.org/topic.cfm?topic=A00389 (accessed March 31, 2009).

———. 2009. Posterior Cruciate Ligament Injuries. AAOS, http://orthoinfo.aaos.org/topic.cfm?topic-A00420 (accessed March 1, 2009).

American Association of Cardiovascular and Pulmonary Rehabilitation (AACVPR). 2006. *AACVPR cardiac rehabilitation resource manual.* Champaign, IL: Human Kinetics.

American College of Sports Medicine. 2010. *Guidelines for exercise testing and prescription.* 8th ed. Philadelphia: Williams and Wilkins.

American Physical Therapy Association. 2008. Physical Therapists Say Appropriate Exercise Can Help Prevent ACL Injuries in Female Athletes. Press Release, http://www.apta.org/AM/Template.cfm?Section=News_Archive&CONTENTID=52503&TEMPLATE=/CM/ContentDisplay.cfm (accessed March 8, 2009).

Arthritis Foundation. 2009. Osteoarthritis Fact Sheet. http://www.arthritis.org/media/newsroom/media-kits/Osteoarthritis_fact_sheet.pdf (accessed March 31, 2009).

Baker, Bradley, and James Lubowitz. 2008. Meniscus Injuries. eMedicine, http://emedicine.medscape.com/article/90661-overview (accessed January 26, 2009).

Birmingham, T., D. Bryant, J. Griffin, R. Litchfield, J. Kramer, A. Donner, and P. Fowler. 2008. A Randomized Controlled Trial Comparing the Effectiveness of Functional Knee Brace and Neoprene Sleeve Use after Anterior Cruciate Ligament Reconstruction. *The American Journal of Sports Medicine* Vol. 36, No. 4: 648–655.

Centers for Disease Control and Prevention. 2008. Alternative Warm-Up Program Reduces Risk of ACL Injuries For Female College Soccer Players: Female Athletes Most at Risk for Ligament Injuries. CDC Press Release, http://www.cdc.gov/media/pressrel/2008/r080725.htm (accessed March 8, 2009).

Christopher, J., M. Wahl, and S. Slaney. 2006. Anterior Cruciate Ligament Tears and Their Treatment: Arthroscopic and Minimally-Invasive Surgery for ACL Reconstruction. UW Medicine: Orthopaedics and Sports Medicine, http://orthop.washington.edu/uw/arthroscopic/tabID_3376/ItemID_289/Articles/Default.aspx (accessed January 20, 2009).

DeBerardino, Thomas, and Jeffrey Gundel. 2006. Medial Collateral Knee Ligament Injury. eMedicine, http://emedicine.medscape.com/article/89890-overview (accessed March 26, 2009).

Ford, K., G. Myer, and T. Hewett. 2003. Valgus Knee Motion During Landing in High School Female and Male Basketball Players. *Medicine and Science in Sports and Exercise* 35: 1745–1750.

Gilchrist, J., B. Mandelbaum, H. Melancon, G. Ryan, H. Silvers, L. Griffin, D. Watanabe, R. Dick, and J. Dvorak. 2008. A Randomized Controlled Trial to Prevent Noncontact Anterior Cruciate Ligament Injury in female Collegiate Soccer Players. *The American Journal of Sports Medicine* Vol. 36, No. 8: 1476–1482.

Griffin, L., M. Albohm, E. Arendt, R. Bahr, B. Beynnon, M. DeMaio, R. Dick, L. Engebretsen, W. Garrett, J. Hannafin, T. Hewett, L. Huston, M. Ireland, R. Johnson, S. Lephart, B. Mandelbaum, B. Mann, P. Marks, S. Marshall, G. Myklebust, F. Noyes, C. Powers, C. Shields, S. Shultz, H. Silvers, J. Slauterbeck, D. Taylor, C. Teitz, E. Wojts, and B. Yu. 2006. Understanding and Preventing Noncontact Anterior Cruciate Ligament Injuries: A Review of the Hunt Valley II Meeting, January 2005. *The American Journal of Sports Medicine* Vol. 34, No. 9: 1512–1532.

Hertling, Darlene, and Randolph M. Kessler. 1996. *Management of Common Musculoskeletal Disorders: Physical Therapy Principles and Methods.* 3rd ed. Philadelphia: Lippincott.

Hewett, T., T. Lindenfeld, J. Riccobene, and F. Noyes. 1999. The Effect of Neuromuscular Training on the Incidence of Knee Injury in Female Athletes: A Prospective Study. *The American Journal of Sports Medicine* Vol. 27, No. 6: 699–706.

Hewett, T. G. Myer, K. Ford, R. Heidt, A. Colosimo, S. McLean, A. van den Bogert, M. Paterno, and P. Succop. 2005. Biomechanical Measures of Neuromuscular Control and Valgus Loading of the Knee Predict Anterior Cruciat Ligament Injury Risk in Female Athletes. *The American Journal of Sports Medicine* Vol. 33, No. 4: 492–501.

Hewett, T., A. Stroupe, T. Nance, and F. Noyes. 1996. Plyometric Training in Female Athletes: Decreased Impact Forces and Increased Hamstring Torques. *The American Journal of Sports Medicine* Vol. 24, No. 6: 765–773.

Hewett, Timothy. 2000. Neuromuscular and Hormonal Factors Associated with Knee Injuries in Female Athletes: Strategies for Intervention. *Sports Medicine* 29 (5): 313–327.

Ho, Sherwin, and Brad Erikson. 2007. Lateral Collateral Knee Ligament Injury. eMedicine, http://emedicine.medscape.com/article/89819-overview (accessed March 1, 2009).

Hubbell, John, and Evan Schwartz. 2006. Anterior Cruciate Ligament Injury. eMedicine, http://emedicine.medscape.com/article/89442-overview (accessed January 26, 2009).

Ingram, J., S. Fields, E. Yard, and R. D. Comstock. 2008. Epidemiology of Knee Injuries Among Boys and Girls in U.S. High School Athletics. *The American Journal of Sports Medicine* 36: 1116–1122.

James, S. L. 1995. Running Injuries to the Knee. *Journal of the American Academy of Orthopaedic Surgeons* Vol. 3: 309–318.

Juhn, Mark. 2009. Patellofemoral Pain Syndrome: A Review and Guidelines for Treatment. American Academy of Family Physicians, http://www.aafp.org/afp/991101ap/2012.html (accessed January 26, 2009).

Kendall, F., E. McCreary, and P. Provance, 1993. *Muscles: Testing and Function.* 4th ed. Baltimore: Williams and Wilkins.

Lutz, G., R. Palmitier, K. An, and E. Chao. 1993. Comparison of Tibiofemoral Joint Forces during Open-Kinetic-Chain and Closed-Kinetic-Chain Exercises. *The Journal of Bone and Joint Surgery* 75: 732–739.

Mandelbaum, B., H. Silvers, D. Watanabe, J. Knarr, S. Thomas, L. Griffin, D. Kirkendall, and W. Garrett. 2005. Effectiveness of a Neuromuscular and Proprioceptive Training Program in Preventing the Incidence of Anterior Cruciate Ligament Injuries in Female Athletes: 2-Year Follow-up. *The American Journal of Sports Medicine* Vol. 33, No. 7: 1–8.

Martinez, J., K. Honsik, and C. Lorenzo. 2009. Iliotibial Band Syndrome. eMedicine http://emidi-cine. medscope.com/article/307850_overview (accessed Sept. 30, 2009).

McDevitt, E., D. Taylor, M. Miller, J. Gerber, G. Ziemke, D. Hinkin, J. Uhovchak, R. Arciero, and P. St. Pierre. 2004. Functional Bracing after Anterior Cruciate Ligament Reconstruction: A Prospective, Randomized Multi-Center Study. *The American Journal of Sports Medicine* Vol. 32, No. 8: 1887-1892.

Moore, Keith L. 1992. *Clinically Oriented Anatomy.* 3rd ed. Baltimore: Williams and Wilkins.

National Collegiate Athletic Association. Female Athletes Found More Susceptible to ACL Injuries. 2009. Interactive Video, http://media.ncaa.org/skins/aclskin/default.aspx?pageid=6c28f11c-85a7-4a22-911d-41e934e98e6b&ss=mediaportal (accessed March 8, 2009).

Norkin, Cynthia C., and Pamela K. Levangie. 1992. *Joint Structure and Function: A Comprehensive Analysis.* 2nd ed. Philadelphia: F.A. Davis Company.

Parolie, J. M., and J. A. Bergfeld. 1986. Long-term Results of Nonoperative Treatment of Isolated Posterior Cruciate Ligament Injuries in the Athlete. *The American Journal of Sports Medicine* 14(1): 35–38.

Peterson, C., T. Agesen, J. Ertl, and G. Kovacs. 2006. Posterior Cruciate Ligament Injury. eMedi-cine, http://emedicine.medscape.com/article/90514-overview (accessed March 1, 2009).

Pettineo, S., K. Jestes, and M. Lehr. 2004. Female ACL Injury Prevention with a Functional Integration Exercise Model. *National Strength and Conditioning Association* Vol. 26, No. 1: 28–33.

Prodromos, C., Y. Han, J. Rogowski, B. Joyce, and K. Shi. 2007. **[Article title?]** *Arthroscopy* 23 (12): 1320–1325.

Santa Monica Orthopaedic and Sports Medicine Group. 2009. ACL Prevention Project. http://www.aclprevent.com (accessed March 1, 2009).

Silvers, Holly, and Bert Mandelbaum. 2007. Prevention of Anterior Cruciate Ligament Injury in the Female Athlete. *British Journal of Sports Medicine* 41: 52–29.

Stensdotter, A., P. Hodges, R. Mellor, G. Sundelin, and C. Hager-Ross. 2003. Quadriceps Activation in Closed and in Open Kinetic Chain Exercise. *Medicine and Science in Sports and Exercise* Vol. 35, No. 12: 2043-3047.

Wright R., and G. Fetzer. 2007. Bracing after ACL Reconstruction: A Systematic Review. *Clinical Orthopaedics and Related Research* 455: 162–168.

About the Author

Erin Erb Hughes, MSPT, C-PT, graduated summa cum laude from Boston University in 1996 with a bachelor of science degree in health studies. In 1998 she completed her master of science degree in physical therapy from the same university. Since that time she has been a practicing physical therapist in Virginia, Maryland, Kansas, and Texas. Erin has worked with a variety of patient populations in numerous settings, including home healthcare, hospital acute care, and outpatient orthopedics. -

Erin has been certified as a personal trainer through the National Strength and Conditioning Association since 2000. In 2002 Erin joined the Desert Southwest Fitness team of course reviewers and is the author of the correspondence courses *Foam Roller Fitness, Exercise for Knee and Hip Replacement, Shoulder Girdle Stabilization,* and the study guide for *Low Back Injury Prevention and Rehab,* published by Desert Southwest Fitness. She has also authored a number of articles for *Advance for Physical Therapists and PTAs.*